Recent Results in Cancer Research 137

F. Raue (Ed.)

Hypercalcemia of Malignancy

With 25 Figures and 17 Tables

Springer-Verlag
Berlin Heidelberg New York
London Paris Tokyo
Hong Kong Barcelona
Budapest

Prof. Dr. F. Raue
Medizinische Universitätsklinik
Innere Medizin I
Bergheimer Straße 58
69115 Heidelberg
Germany

ISBN-13: 978-3-642-85075-2 e-ISBN-13: 978-3-642-85073-8
DOI: 10.1007/978-3-642-85073-8

CIP data applied for

Softcover reprint of the hardcover 1st edition 1994

Typesetting: Best-set Typesetter Ltd., Hong Kong
SPIN: 10128559 19/3130/SPS – 5 4 3 2 1 0 – Printed on acid-free paper

Contents

*List of Contributors**

---

* The address of the principal author is given on the first page of each contribution.
[1] Page on which contribution begins.

Biological Aspects

Cytokines as Mediators of Hypercalcemia of Malignancy

J. Pfeilschifter

Department of Internal Medicine I, – Endocrinology and Metabolism, University of Heidelberg, Bergheimerstraße 58, 69115 Heidelberg, Germany

Hypercalcemia of malignancy is due to the breakdown of the normal regulation of calcium homeostasis. It is caused by an abnormally large production of one or several cytokines and/or other regulatory factors by the tumor cells capable of influencing the effectors of calcium homeostasis. There is little doubt that calcium release from bone contributes greatly to the hypercalcemia seen with humoral hypercalcemia of malignancy. Bone resorption is also certainly the major contributing factor in the hypercalcemia observed with many hematologic diseases or local bone metastases. In this chapter I will focus on the role of cytokines in this type of tumor-increased bone resorption, although one should be fully aware that increased calcium reabsorption from the kidney or increased calcium absorption from the intestinal tract may contribute to a variable degree to the whole picture of hypercalcemia of malignancy.

Tumor-Induced Bone Resorption Is Osteoclast Mediated

Bone is constantly remodeled throughout life. Calcium release occurs during the resorption of bone by multinucleated osteoclasts through acidification of a tightly sealed space between the osteoclast surface and the bone surface. Although there is some in vitro evidence that tumor cells themselves may lyse bone by direct proteolytic effects (Eilon and Mundy 1978), the majority of bone loss seems to be mediated through an increase in osteoclastic bone resorption, as judged from the increased numbers of osteoclasts in histologic samples from patients with hypercalcemia of malignancy (Galasko 1976; Steward et al. 1982).

Which Are the Mediators of the Tumor-Induced Increases in Osteoclasts?

Increased osteoclastic activity as a result of the presence of a tumor implies that the tumor cells must secrete one or several agents capable of stimulating osteoclast generation or function. These tumor products may be circulating systemically or be locally produced by tumor cells within the bone marrow in such quantities that local and systemic regulatory mechanisms of osteoclastic resorption and calcium homeostasis are being overwhelmed. As a consequence, hypercalcemia results.

Nearly all major classic hormones are capable of affecting the rate of osteoclast formation and activity. Among them are parathyroid hormone (PTH), 1,25-dihydroxyvitamin D_3, calcitonin, estrogens, glucocorticoids, and thyroid hormones (Mundy 1989). Indeed, we know many clinical syndromes where an unbalanced increase in the concentration of these classical hormones causes hypercalcemia, such as with PTH in primary hyperparathyroidism or with 1,25-dihydroxyvitamin D_3 in sarcoidosis. Nevertheless, with the exception of certain lymphomas, these hormones are only rarely produced by malignant tumors (Yoshimoto et al. 1989; Nussbaum et al. 1990) and they do not appear to be the predominant mediators of hypercalcemia of malignancy. Often their serum levels are rather downregulated in an attempt to counterbalance the increased bone resorption (Steward et al. 1980; Ralston et al. 1984).

Cytokine Network

When therefore during the last 2 decades another class of hormone-like polypeptides appeared that seemed to be produced in abundant amounts by tumor cells and many of whose members had profound stimulatory effects on bone resorption in vitro, many researchers had the feeling that the mediators of hypercalcemia of malignancy had finally been found. These agents have been grouped together sometimes arbitrarily as lymphokines and growth factors, although the distinction between the different groups of these polypeptides has vanished with time. In the following text I will therefore rather use the global term "cytokine," to summarize them. The list of peptide cytokines is ever increasing and today holds more than 50 different species and subspecies some of which may be grouped in larger families.

Just like the classic hormones, most cytokines are secreted in a regulated fashion from cells, bind to specific target receptors and use similar intracellular signal transmission pathways (Sporn and Roberts 1990). Many cytokines appear to have only a short range of action which restricts their effects to the tissue where they are produced. Nevertheless, as I will discuss below, there is more and more evidence that some cytokines may also have systemic effects if only produced in large enough amounts. The one major difference between the classic hormones and the various cytokines, however, appears to be the rather restricted expression of the classic hormones, whereas most cytokines are expressed in a large variety of tissues (Sporn and Roberts 1990).

There are many interactions between hormones and cytokines. Hormone release is regulated by cytokines in most glands, and hormonal effects on target tissues are often mediated or modified by the secondary release of cytokines produced in the target tissues. This also appears to be true for bone, where the effects of PTH have been shown to be partially mediated by the cytokine insulin-like growth factor I (IGF-I) (Canalis et al. 1989), and estrogens seem to exert their suppressive effects on bone resorption through the inhibition of resorption-stimulating cytokines, such as interleukin-1, 6, and tumor necrosis factor (Horowitz 1993).

Cytokine Effects on Bone Resorption

Most of the known cytokines whose actions have been examined in one of the in vitro models of bone tissue have been observed to have some effect on the proliferation or function of bone cells. Many of them are indeed locally produced by bone cells and seem to be essential for the local regulation of bone turnover (Pfeilschifter et al. 1990).

Bone resorption is dependent on the continuous generation of new osteoclasts from hematopoietic precursor cells. The multiple steps of osteoclast development offer ample possibilities of control through cytokines. In fact, cytokines are involved in the control of proliferation of still pluripotent stem cells and affect the differentiation of these cells, they control the fusion of the committed precursor cells, their movement towards the bone surface, the attachment of mature osteoclasts to the bone surface and their bone-resorbing activity (Mundy and Roodman 1987).

Table 1 lists the cytokines currently known to stimulate either osteoclast precursor proliferation and/or activity of mature osteoclasts. Not all of these cytokines may act directly on the osteoclast. There is good evidence that many potent cytokine stimulators of bone resorption act primarily via the osteoblasts or other mesenchymal bone marrow cells. The primary target cell then releases a secondary mediator capable of stimulating osteoclast proliferation or activity (see also Fig. 1). One of these classes of mediators seem to be the prostaglandins since addition of indomethacin in vitro often blocks the bone-resorbing affect of cytokines (Tashjian and Levine 1978; Tashjian et al. 1982, 1985, 1987). However, there also appear to be other classes of secondary mediators whose structure still has to be elucidated (Rodan and Martin 1981).

It is difficult to place all cytokines capable of directly or indirectly stimulating bone resorption in distinct groups according to their actions since many of their effects seem to overlap. Some of them, such as IGF-I, platelet-derived growth factor (PDGF), fibroblast growth factor (FGF), or epidermal growth factor (EGF), appear to have a general stimulatory effect on proliferation in many cell types and may thus be rather nonselective "growth factors." Others such as the colony-stimulating factors (CSF), stem

Table 1. Cytokines that cause increased osteoclastic bone resorption

Cytokine	Increased proliferation of precursor cells	Increased activity of mature cells
Stem cell factor (SCF)	Demulder et al. 1992	
Macrophage colony-stimulating factor (M-CSF)	MacDonald et al. 1986 Yoshida et al. 1990 Takahashi et al. 1991 Corboz et al. 1992 Tanaka et al. 1993 Orcel et al. 1993	
Granulocyte macrophage colony-stimulating factor (GM-CSF)	MacDonald et al. 1986 Takahashi et al. 1991	
Leukocyte inhibitory factor (LIF)	Reid et al. 1990 Lowe et al. 1991	Reid et al. 1990 Lowe et al. 1991
Interleukin 1 (IL-1)	Pfeilschifter et al. 1989	Gowen et al. 1983 Thomson et al. 1986
Interleukin 3 (IL-3)	Barton and Mayer 1989 Takahashi et al. 1991	
Interleukin 6 (IL-6)	Kurihara et al. 1990 Jilka et al. 1992	
Interleukin 11 (IL-11)	Passeri et al. 1992	
Tumor necrosis factor (TNF)	Pfeilschifter et al. 1988	Bertolini et al. 1986 Tashjian et al. 1987 Thomson et al. 1987
Epidermal growth factor (EGF)	Raisz et al. 1980	Tashjian and Levine 1978
Fibroblast growth factor (FGF)	Simmons and Raisz 1991	Shen et al. 1989
Insulin-like growth factor I (IGF-I)	Ibbotson et al. 1992 Mochizuki et al. 1992 Slootweg et al. 1992	
PTH-related peptide (PTHrP)		Yates et al. 1988 Steward et al. 1988
Platelet-derived growth factor (PDGF)		Tashjian et al. 1982 Cochran et al. 1993
Transforming growth factor alpha (TGF-α)	Ibbotson et al. 1985b Takahashi et al. 1986	Tashjian et al. 1985
Transforming growth factor β (TGF-β)		Tashjian et al. 1985 Pfeilschifter et al. 1988 Dieudonne et al. 1991

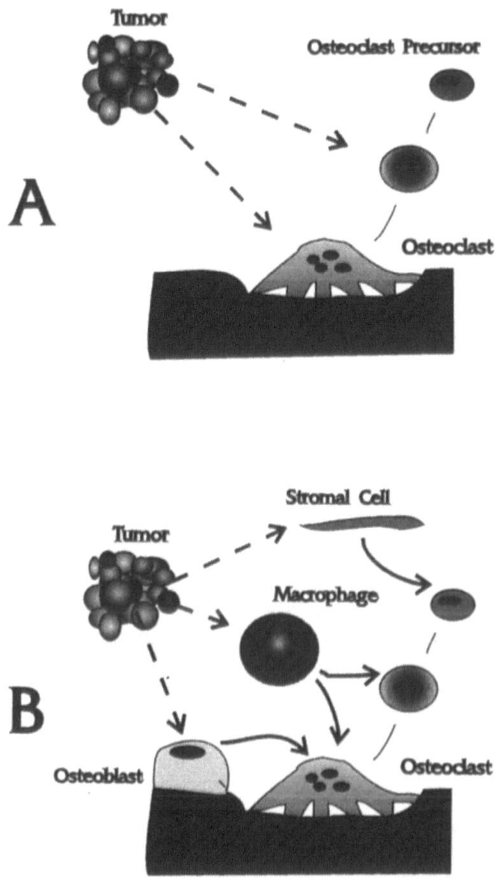

Fig. 1A,B. Potential mechanisms of action of tumor products on osteoclast generation and function. **A** Direct stimulatory effect on osteoclast precursors and/or mature osteoclasts. **B** Indirect stimulatory effects through local osteoblasts, other mesenchymal stroma cells, or macrophages

cell factor (SCF), leukocyte inhibitory factor (LIF) or interleukin 6 (IL-6) have prominent affects on the maturation of marrow cells and seem to influence bone resorption predominantly by their effects on hematopoietic precursor cells including osteoclast precursors.

We also know a limited number of counterregulatory factors capable of decreasing osteoclast development, which in vivo seem to balance the stimulatory effects of the above-mentioned cytokines (Table 2). Among them are interleukin-4 (IL-4) and endothelin, transforming growth factor β (TGF-β), and members of the related bone morphogenetic protein (BMP) family. TGF-β has complicated affects on bone resorption, depending on the stage of osteoclastic maturation and the bone environment (Tables 1, 2).

Table 2. Cytokines that cause decreased osteoclastic bone resorption

Cytokine	Decreased proliferation of precursor cells	Decreased activity of mature cells
Osteoinductive factor (OIF)	Kukita et al. 1990	Oreffo et al. 1990
Transforming growth factor β (TGF-β)	Chenu et al. 1988 Dieudonne et al. 1991	Oreffo et al. 1990
Endothelin-1	Alam et al. 1992	
Interleukin 4 (IL-4)	Watanabe et al. 1990 Shioi et al. 1991	
PTH-related peptide (PTHrP) Carboxy-terminal peptide	Fenton et al. 1991 Fenton et al. 1993	

Although we know from animal mutation models that some of these cytokines such as macrophage-CSF are essential for the orderly generation of osteoclasts (Wiktor-Jedrzejczak et al. 1990), we still know little about the relative importance of each cytokine in normal bone turnover and how they are regulated in bone. Specific binding proteins, proteases, control by other cytokines and by systemic hormones all appear to be important aspects of their regulation (Nathan and Sporn 1991).

Evidence for Cytokine Involvement in Humoral Hypercalcemia of Malignancy

In humoral hypercalcemia of malignancy (HHM), bone resorption is stimulated by a malignant tumor which has not invaded the bone and is not in direct contact with the skeleton. Thus some factor produced by the tumor cells must have a hormone-like action on bone resorption. Given the capability of many cytokines to stimulate bone resorption and their release in large amounts from many tumors – some are probably necessary for the maintenance of the neoplastic phenotype – it was tempting to speculate that some of them may be mediators of tumor hypercalcemia. In order to find cytokines that may contribute to the humoral type of hypercalcemia, two lines of evidence had to be pursued:

1. The implicated cytokine should account for most or all of the bone-resorbing activity of the tumor.
2. The cytokine must be capable of exerting systemic effects on bone metabolism.

Just as any normal cell, a tumor cell usually produces a variety of cytokines. To pick out the cytokine that may be involved in the hypercalcemic effect researchers looked for those cytokines with a major bone-resorbing effect in vitro by biochemical or immunologic analysis. This would then appear to be the best candidate for the hypercalcemic effect in vivo. Thus, Ibbotson et al. (1985a) demonstrated that antibodies against the EGF receptor (which is identical with the TGF-α receptor) could completely abolish bone-resorbing activity in vitro in a solid tumor producing TGF-α, making TGF-α a strong candidate for the bone-resorbing effect of this tumor in vivo. A similar inhibition of bone resorptive activity with specific antibodies has been shown with a tumor model producing IL-1 activity (Sato et al. 1987).

Although these data provide strong circumstantial evidence for the role of these cytokines as mediators of hypercalcemia of malignancy, one should point out some of the problems with this in vitro approach:

1. All in vitro resorption models are limited in their usefulness for predicting bone resorption in vivo. Often they reflect only part of the osteoclast generation or only the activity of mature osteoclasts (Pfeilschifter et al. 1988).
2. As already mentioned above, the agents produced by the tumor cells may not even necessarily directly affect the osteoclasts but rather affect them indirectly via mesenchymal cells or macrophages (Fig. 1). This kind of mechanism may go undetected in the organ culture bone resorption assays since the composition of the cell types in vitro may not accurately reflect the composition of cell types in vivo. Indeed, Yoneda et al. (1989) showed that, in mice bearing MH-85 tumor cells, TNF was increased fourfold in plasma, and hypercalcemia could be reduced by antibodies to TNF, although the tumor cells did not appear to produce TNF themselves. Rather the tumor cells appeared to stimulate TNF production by the host-immune cells.

As mentioned above, cytokines are rather locally active agents that often have a short range of action. Thus, not all cytokines capable of stimulating bone resorption in vitro may be good candidates for having systemic effects on bone resorption in vivo. Nevertheless a couple of cytokines when injected or overexpressed in vivo have been demonstrated to be capable of inducing hypercalcemia, including PTH-related peptide (PTHrP) (Steward et al. 1988; Yates et al. 1988), TGF-α (Tsashjian et al. 1986; Yates et al. 1992), TNF (Johnson et al. 1989), IL-1 (Sabatini et al. 1988), IL-6 (Black et al. 1991), EGF (Tashjian et al. 1986), and LIF (Cornish et al. 1993). All of these cytokines therefore appear to be potential candidates for mediators of HHM (Table 3).

PTHrP as the Major Mediator of HHM

Although many of the cytokines listed in Table 1 appear to be good potential candidates for mediators of HHM, strictly convincing evidence for their role in HHM has so far only been produced for one cytokine: the PTH-related

Table 3. Mediators of hypercalcemia of malignancy

Humoral hypercalcemia of malignancy (HHM)	PTHrP (other cytokines?)
Multiple myeloma	TNF IL-1 IL-6
Lymphoma	PTHrP TNF 1,25-Vitamin D_3
Bone metastases	(Various cytokines?)

peptide (PTHrP). In fact, in contrast to all other cytokines, this particular cytokine was discovered through its hypercalcemic actions in HHM, emphasizing its crucial role in HHM (Moseley et al. 1987; Suva et al. 1987; Martin et al. 1989). PTHrP seems to be the single most important mediator of HHM for the majority of solid tumors such as squamous cell carcinoma of the lung, head and neck, and carcinoma of the kidney, the ovary, and the pancreas (Mundy and Martin 1982). It fulfils both premises listed above, i.e., it is the major bone-resorbing cytokine produced by many tumors, and it can reproduce the humoral hypercalcemia of malignancy syndrome in vitro and in vivo (Kemp et al. 1988; Horiuchi et al. 1988; Yates et al. 1988; Sartori et al. 1988; Pizurki et al. 1988; Steward et al. 1988, 1989; Thorikay et al. 1989). Moreover, in animal models of HHM the biochemical abnormalities can be completely corrected by infusion of antisera against PTH-rP (Kukreja et al. 1988, 1990; Henderson et al. 1990a). Most important, elevated levels of this cytokine can be detected in the vast majority of solid tumors causing HHM (Burtis et al. 1990; Henderson et al. 1990b).

It is interesting to note that PTHrP, as the name implies, shares its receptor with the classic hormone PTH (Caulfield et al. 1990), a fact which – with the exception of insulin and the insulin-like growth factors – appears to be rather unique for a cytokine and may indicate its intermediate role between a systemic hormone and a local cytokine. Nevertheless, PTHrP appears to be expressed in many tissues including bone (Kramer et al. 1991; Bergmann et al. 1990) and there act as a local regulator just like any other cytokine, which makes it a true member of the cytokine family. Its role in normal bone metabolism appears to be even more complicated by the recently discovered fact that a carboxy-teminal fragment of PTHrP turns out to be an inhibitor rather than a stimulator of bone resorption (Fenton et al. 1991, 1993). Since the occurrence, properties, and functions of this protein are discussed at length in Chap. 2 of this volume, I will restrain at this point from going into more detail concerning this cytokine.

Are There Other Cytokine Mediators of HHM?

There appears to be a minority of tumors where hypercalcemia cannot be explained by increased PTHrP production. It is quite possible that IL-1, TNF, or TGF-α, as already mentioned above, and 1,25-dihydroxyvitamin D_3 (Yamanoto et al. 1987) are involved in these cases.

Even when observed at an elevated concentration in HHM, PTHrP may not be the sole mediator of hypercalcemia. There is good in vivo evidence that PTHrP infusions together with a potent bone-resorbing cytokine such as IL-1 can potentiate hypercalcemia produced by each agent alone, which makes it possible that other cytokines may at least partially contribute to the hypercalcemic effects (Sato et al. 1989). Moreover, it has been a long-standing observation that bone formation in most patients with HHM is rather depressed (McDonell et al. 1982; Steward et al. 1982), a finding that may not be easily reconciled with the effects of PTHrP alone. In primary hyperparathyroidism, the excess PTH which shares its receptor with PTHrP rather increases bone formation. Indeed, most other cytokines such as TNF or IL-1 that would be eligible as other candidates for HHM depress bone formation in vitro (Pfeilschifter et al. 1990). Another puzzling finding is that of depressed 1,25-dihydroxyvitamin D_3 levels in many patients with HHM (Steward et al. 1980), despite the fact that PTHrP stimulates the renal 1-α-hydroxylase activity. This may also point to additional factors besides PTHrP being responsible for the whole picture of HHM. The measurement of other cytokines in patients with HHM and the use of neutralizing antibodies in in vivo experiments may eventually clarify the role of such cosecreted cytokines.

Cytokines as Mediators of Bone Resorption in Multiple Myeloma

Unlike in solid tumors, PTHrP does not seem to play a major role in hypercalcemia caused by multiple myeloma. Hypercalcemia due to bone destruction occurs in between 20% and 40% of all patients with multiple myeloma at some time during the course of the disease. It has been perceived for a long time that myeloma cells produce cytokines capable of stimulating osteoclastic bone resorption (Mundy et al. 1974; Mundy and Bertolini 1986). In some myeloma cultures tumor necrosis factor β (TNFβ), also termed lymphotoxin, was observed to be the predominant bone-resorbing cytokine (Garrett et al. 1987). Other bone-resorbing cytokines, such as interleukin 1 and 6, are also produced by myeloma cells (Bataille et al. 1989; Kawano et al. 1989; Cozzolino et al. 1989), and may also be involved in increased bone resorption in multiple myeloma. Kawano et al. (1989) examined four cultures of myeloma whose bone-resorbing activity in vitro seemed to be entirely due to IL-1β as judged from antibody-blocking experiments.

Although these data do not strictly prove that TNFβ, IL-1, and IL-6 are indeed responsible for the increased resorption in myeloma, they are as good circumstantial evidence as there is today. Neutralization of the tumor products in vivo by specific antibodies to obtain further proof may be even more difficult to achieve in this type of tumor due to the local effect of the cytokines involved.

Malignant Lymphomas

Patients with lymphomas only occasionally develop hypercalcemia (Canellos 1974). Hypercalcemia has been described in patients with Hodgkin's disease, B-cell lymphomas, T-cell lymphomas, and Burkitt's lymphoma. In some of these patients increased production of 1,25-dihydroxyvitamin D_3 by lymphoma cells may be involved in the pathogenesis of the hypercalcemia (Breslau et al. 1984; Rosenthal et al. 1985; Jacobson et al. 1989; Scheinman et al. 1991). Thus hypercalcemia in these lymphomas resembles the hypercalcemia that occurs in granulomatous benign disordes such as sarcoidosis. TNFβ has been observed to be increased in the serum from patients with adult T-cell lymphoma who were hypercalcemic, but not in normocalcemic patients, and calcium levels were positively correlated with the TNF concentrations, indicating a role for this cytokine in the pathogenesis of hypercalcemia in some cases (Matsuda et al. 1990; Ishibashi et al. 1991). Lymphomas in the dog associated with hypercalcemia seem to be associated with increased circulating concentrations of PTHrP but these levels do not seem to correlate well with hypercalcemia (Rosol et al. 1992).

Hypercalcemia with Osteolytic Metastases

Apart from PTHrP, tumor cells of bone metastases may also secrete short-ranging cytokines that may induce or enhance bone resorption. The most common cause in this group of cancers is breast cancer. Whereas in 65% of these patients hypercalcemia seems to be due to systemically active PTHrP secreted by the tumor cells (Grill et al. 1991), the others seem to have local mechanisms involved. Hypercalcemia due to lytic bone metastases appears late in the course of the disease and requires extensive metastatic disease. Breast cancer cells produce a variety of cytokines (Salomon et al. 1984) and all cytokines mentioned in Table 1 may in fact be candidates for causing hypercalcemia in bone metastasis.

Mechanisms of Hypercalcemia Not Related to Increased Bone Resorption or Due to Secondary Causes

In many cases, coexisting underlying conditions such as primary hyperparathyroidism, sarcoidosis, immobilization or hypercalcemia-inducing medications may the cause of the hypercalcemia.

It is also important to point out that the hypercalcemia mediated by PTHrP is only partially mediated by increased bone resorption. At least some of the hypercalcemic action may be explained by the effect of PTHrP on the kidney, i.e., increased tubular calcium reabsorption (Steward et al. 1980). Indeed, serum calcium levels often do not closely reflect increases in bone resorption (Harinck et al. 1987), but may also be influenced by impaired glomerular filtration. These two effects can be dissociated by using bisphosphonates as potent inhibitors of bone resorption. At least a partial lowering effect on serum calcium can be observed in all cases. In many patients even a complete normalization can be achieved. Nevertheless, in some patients, a residual amount of hypercalcemia seems to be due to a nephrogenic mechanism (Hutardo et al. 1991; Grill et al. 1992). Nephrogenic mechanisms may certainly also play a role in hypercalcemia with multiple myeloma due to immunoglobulin light chain deposition (Durie et al. 1981). Rare cases of hypercalcemia of malignancy may be due to increased absorption of calcium from the intestinal tract (Doppelt et al. 1982).

On the Specificity of Cytokines Involved in Hypercalcemia of Malignancy

When the cytokine class was discovered it was intriguing to speculate on this class of polypepetides being involved in the mechanisms of hypercalcemia of malignancy since most tumors produce a variety of these cytokines and, as mentioned above, many cytokines have bone-resorbing effects in vitro and in vivo. As it turned out, this class of peptides indeed seemed to provide the answer to the mechanism of hypercalcemia in many, if not most, cases of malignant tumors. With our increasing knowledge about cytokines this seems to be more astonishing today than it may have seemed a couple of years ago.

In fact, none of the cytokines implicated in hypercalcemia of malignancy so far is specific for bone. Moreover, up to the present day, no cytokine involved in hypercalcemia has been discovered that may be a specific tumor cell product. All of the implicated cytokines, including PTHrP, interleukins 1 and 6, and TNF are also produced in a large variety of cell types outside bone and have characteristic effects on many tissues totally unrelated to bone resorption.

Nevertheless, one has to make the assumption that a massive and unregulated secretion of these cytokines may be sufficient in overwhelming controlled bone resorption and cause hypercalcemia. This may indeed seem surprising since, as judged from immunohistologic evidence, production of PTHP in normal skin alone should easily surpass total production of PTH (Atillasoy et al. 1991). However, it might be possible that the tumor cell environment faciltitates the escape of these cytokines into the circulation which might normally be locally contained, or alternatively there may be subtle changes in posttranscriptional modifications of these mediators in the tumor environment that might make them more available as systemic mediators. In the case of local metastases, the same cytokines released from metastases in bone causing increased bone resorption may have quite different effects when released from metastases settled in another tissue.

Given the global role of these cytokines as regulators of cell function and the variety of effects they produce in vitro (Sporn and Roberts 1988), it may also seem surprising that overproduction of one or more of these regulators in HHM may simply result in a stimulation of bone resorption in vivo without other major "side effects." This may, however, just be a question of the affinity of a cytokine for different cell types as well as the sensitivity of different types of cells, and applies in a similar fashion to the uncontrolled production of classic hormones.

Clinical Implications Derived from the Pathophysiologic Data

Is anything that we have learned so far about the role of cytokines in hypercalcemia of malignancy useful for patient management?

First of all the knowledge about likely mediators and the increasing capability of measuring them in serum may provide us with a better means to differentiate HHM from different causes of hypercalcemia and may help in quickly elucidating a definite diagnosis, since a tumor is often not evident when hypercalcemia occurs.

Second, these cytokines may prove valuable as markers for monitoring tumor burden before and after treatment procedures even in those cases where the amount of cytokines released from the tumor may not sufficiently increase bone resorption to raise serum calcium levels.

Third, in the long run, knowledge of these cytokines may prove valuable in designing specific antagonists against them or against their receptors, which would be the most rational approach against tumor-associated hypercalcemia. Given the options of potent agents such as the bisphosphonates as inhibitors of tumor-mediated bone resorption which are presented in more detail in Chap. 9, this may still be a distant prospect, but these antagonists may be most valuable in those cases where the cytokine not only affects bone resorption but also kidney function.

References

Alam ASMT, Gallagher A, Shankar V, Ghatei MA, Datta HK, Huang L-H, Moonga BS, Chambers TJ, Bloom SR, Zaidi M (1992) Endothelin inhibits osteoclastic bone resorption by a direct effect on cell motility: implications for the vascular control of bone resorption. Endocrinology 130:3617–3624

Atillasoy EJ, Burtis WJ, Milstone LM (1991) Immunohistochemical localization of parathyroid hormone-related protein (PTHrP) in normal human skin. J Invest Dermatol 96:277–280

Barton BE, Mayer R (1989) IL-3 induces differentiation of bone marrow precursor cells to osteoclast-like cells. J Immunol 143:3211–3216
Bataille R, Jourdan M, Zhang X-G, Klein B (1989) Serum levels of interleukin-6, a potent myeloma cell growth factor, as a reflection of disease severity in plasma cell dyscrasias. J Clin Invest 84:2008–2011
Bergmann P, Nijs-De Wof N, Pepersack T, Corvilain J (1990) Release of parathyroid hormone-like pepetides by fetal rat long bones in culture. J Bone Miner Res 7:741–753
Bertolini DR, Nedwin GR, Bringman TS, Smith DD, Mundy GR (1986) Stimulation of bone resorption and inhibition of bone formation in vitro by hyman tumor necrosis factors. Nature 319:516
Black K, Garrett IR, Mundy GR (1991) Chinese hamster ovarian cells transfected with the murine interleukin-6 gene cause hypercalcemia as well as cachexia, leukocytosis and thrombocytosis in tumor-bearing nude mice. Endocrinology 128:2657–2659
Breslau NA, McGuire JL, Zerwekh JE, Frenkel EP, Pak CYC (1984) Hypercalcemia associated with increased serum calcitriol levels in three patients with lymphoma. Ann Intern Med 100:1–7
Burtis WJ, Brady TG, Orloff JJ, Ersbak JB,Warrell RP, Olson BR, Wu TL, Mitnick ME, Broadus AE, Steward AE (1990) Immunochemical characterization of circulating parathyroid hormone-related protein in patients with humoral hypercalcemia of cancer. N Engl J Med 322:1106–1112
Canalis E, Centrella M, Burch W, McCarthy TL (1989) Insulin-like growth factor 1 mediates selective anabolic effects of parathyroid hormone in bone cultures. J Clin Invest 83:60–65
Canellos GP (1974) Hypercalcemia in malignant lymphoma and leukemia. Ann NY Acad Sci 230:240–246
Caulfield MP, McKee RL, Goldman ME, Thiede MA, Thompson DD, Fisher JE (1990) Parathyroid hormone-related protein (PTHrP). Studies with synthetic peptides indicate that parathyroid hormone and PTHrP interact with the same receptor. Nucl Med Biol 17:633–637
Chenu C, Pfeilschifter J, Mundy GR, Roodman GD (1988) Transforming growth factor β inhibits formation of osteoclast-like cells in long-term human marrow culture. Proc Natl Acad Sci USA 85:5682–5687
Cochran DL, Rouse CA, Lynch SE, Graves DT (1993) Effects of platelet-derived growth factor isoforms on calcium release from neonatal mouse calvariae. Bone 14:53–58
Corboz VA, Cecchini MG, Felix R, Fleisch H, van der Pluijm G, Löwik CWGM (1992) Effect of macrophage colony-stimulating factor on in vitro osteoclast generation and bone resorption. Endocrinology 130:437–442
Cornish J, Callon K, Edgar S, Reid IR (1993) The effect of leukemia inhibitory factor on bone in vivo. Endocrinology 132:1359–1366
Cozzolino F, Torcia M, Aldinucci D, Rubartelli A, Miliani A, Shaw AR, Lansdorp PM, Di Gugliemo R (1989) Production of interleukin-1 by bone marrow myeloma cells. Blood 74:3817–387
Demulder A, Suggs SV, Zsebo KM, Scarcez T, Roodman GD (1992) Effects of stem cell factor on osteoclast-like cell formation in long-term human marrow cultures. J Bone Miner Res 7:1337–1344
Dieudonne SC, Foo P, van Zoelen EJJ, Burger EH (1991) Inhibiting and stimulating effects of TGF-β1 on osteoclastic bone resorption in fetal mouse bone organ cultures. J Bone Miner Res 6:479–487
Doppelt SH, Slovik DM, Neer RM, Nolan J, Zusman RM, Potts JT (1982) Gut-mediated hypercalcemia in rabbits bearing VX2 carcinoma: new mechanism for tumor-induced hypercalcemia. Proc Natl Acad Sci USA 79:640–644

Durie BGM, Salmon SE, Mundy GR (1981) Relation of osteoclast activating factor production to the extent of metastatic bone disease in myeloma. Br J Haematol 47:21–30
Eilon G, Mundy GR (1978) Direct resorption of bone by human breast cancer cells in vitro. Nature 276:726–728
Fenton AJ, Kemp BE, Kent GN, Moseley JM, Zheng M-H, Rowe DJ, Britto JM, Martin TJ, Nicholson GC (1991) A carboxy-terminal peptide from the parathyroid hormone-related protein inhibits bone resorption by osteoclasts. Endocrinology 129:1762–1768
Fenton AJ, Martin TJ, Nicholson GC (1993) Long-term culture of disaggregated rat osteoclasts: inhibition of bone resorption and reduction of osteoclast-like cell number by calcitonin and PTHrP[107-139]. J Cell Physiol 155:1–7
Galasko CSB (1976) Mechanisms of bone destruction in the development of skeletal metastases. Nature 263:507–508
Garrett RI, Durie BGM, Nedwin GE, Gillespie A, Bringman T, Sabatini M, Bertolini DR, Mundy GR (1987) Production of the bone resorbing cytokine lymphotoxin by cultured human myeloma cells. N Engl J Med 317:526–532
Gowen M, Wood DD, Ihrie EJ, McGuire MKB, Russell RGG (1983) An interleukin 1 like factor stimulates bone resorption in vitro. Nature 306:378–380
Grill V, Ho P, Moseley JM, Johanson N, Lee S, Body J, Kukreja S, Martin TJ (1991) Parathyroid hormone-related protein: elevated levels both in human hypercalcemia of malignancy and in hypercalcemia complicating metastatic breast cancer. J Clin Endocrinol Metab 73:1309–1315
Grill V, Murray RML, Ho PWM, Santamaria JD, Pitt P, Potts C, Jerums G, Martin TJ (1992) Circulating PTH and PTH-rP levels before and after treatment of tumor induced hypercalcemia with pamidronate disodium (APD). J Clin Endocrinol Metab 74:1468–1470
Harinck HIJ, Bijvoet OLM, Platingh AST (1987) Role of bone and kidney in tumor-induced hypercalcemia and its treatment with bisphosphonates and sodium chloride. Am J Med 82:1133–1142
Henderson J, Bernier S, D'Amour P, Goltzman D (1990a) Effects of passive immunization against parathyroid hormone (PTH)-like peptide and PTH in hypercalcemic tumor-bearing rats and normocalcemic controls. Endocrinology 127:1310–1318
Henderson JE, Shustik C, Kremer R, Rabbani SA, Hendy GN, Goltzman D (1990b) Circulating concentrations of parathyroid hormone-like peptide in malignancy and in hyperparathyroidism. J Bone Miner Res 5:105–113
Horiuchi N, Caulfield MD, Fisher JE, Goldman ME, McKnee RL, Reagan JE, Levy JJ, Nutt RF, Rodan SB, Schofield TL, Clemens TL, Rosenblatt M (1988) Similarity of synthetic peptide from human tumor to PTH in vivo and in vitro. Science 238:1566–1568
Horowitz MC (1993) Cytokines and estrogen in bone: anti-osteoporotic effects. Science 260:626–227
Hutardo J, Esbrit P, Rapado A (1991) Relative role of bone and kidney in the hypercalcemia associated with the rat walker carcinosarcoma 256. Eur J Cancer 27:76–79
Ibbotson KJ, D'Souza SM, Smith DD, Carpenter G, Mundy GR (1985a) EGF receptor antiserum inhibits bone resorbing activity produced by a rat Leydig cell tumor associated with the humoral hypercalcemia of malignancy. Endocrinology 116:469–471
Ibbotson KJ, Twardzik DR, D'Souza SM, Hargreaves WR, Todaro GJ, Mundy GR (1985b) Stimulation of bone resorption in vitro by synthetic transforming growth factor-alpha. Science 228:1007–1009

Ibbotson KJ, Orcutt CM, D'Souza SM, Paddock CL, Arthur JA, Jankowsky ML, Boyce RW (1992) Contrasting effects of parathyroid hormone and insulin-like growth factor I in an aged ovariectomized rat model of postmenopausal osteoporosis. J Bone Miner Res 7:425–432.

Ishibashi K, Ishitsuka K, Chuman Y, Otsuka M, Kuwazura Y, Iwahashi M, Utsunomiya A, Hanada S, Sakurami T, Arima T (1991) Tumor necrosis factor-β in the serum of adult T-cell leukemia with hypercalcemia. Blood 77:2451–2455

Jacobson JO, Bringhurst FR, Harris NL, Weitzman SA, Aisenberg AC (1989) Humoral hypercalcemia in Hodgin's disease clinical and laboratory evaluation. Cancer 63:917–923

Jilka RL, Hangoc G, Girasole G, Passeri G, Williams DC, Abrams JS, Boyce B, Broxmeyer H, Manolagas SC (1992) Increased osteoclast development after estrogen loss: mediation by interleukin-6. Science 257:88–91

Johnson RA, Boyce BF, Mundy GR, Roodman GD (1989) Tumors producing human tumor necrosis factor induce hypercalcemia and osteoclastic bone resorption in nude mice. Endocrinology 124:1424–1427

Kawano M, Yamamoto I, Iwato K, Tanaka H, Asaoku H, Tanabe O, Ishikawa H, Nabuyoshi M, Ohmoto Y, Hirai Y, Kuramoto A (1989) Interleukin-1 beta rather than lymphotoxin as the major bone resorbing activity in human multiple myeloma. Blood 73:1646–1649

Kemp BE, Moseley JM, Rodda CP, Ebeling PR, Wettenhall REH, Stapleton D, Dieffenbacher-Jagger H, Ure F, Michelangeli VP, Simmons HA, Raisz LG, Martin TJ (1988) PTH-related protein of malignancy: active synthetic fragments. Science 238:1568–1570

Kramer S, Reynolds FH, Castillo M, Valenzuela DM, Thorikay M, Sorvillo JM (1991) Immunological identification and distribution of parathyroid hormone-related protein in normal and malignant tissues. Endocrinology 128:1927–1937

Kukita A, Bonewald L, Rosen D, Seyedin S, Mundy GR, Roodman GD (1990) Osteoinductive factor inhibits formation of human osteoclast-like cells. Proc Natl Acad Sci USA 87:3023–3026

Kukreja SC, Shevrin DH, Wimbricus SA, Ebeling PR, Danks JA, Rodda CP, Wood WI, Martin TJ (1988) Antibodies to parathyroid hormone-related protein lower serum calcium in athymic mouse models of malignancy-associated hypercalcemia due to human tumors. J Clin Invest 82:1798–1802

Kukreja SC, Rosol TJ, Wimbicus SA, Shevrin DH, Grill V, Barengolts EI, Martin TJ (1990) Tumor resection and antibodies to parathyroid hormone-related protein cause similar changes on bone histomorphometry in hypercalcemia of cancer. Endocrinology 127:305–310

Kurihara N, Bertolini D, Suda T, Akiyama Y, Roodman GD (1990) IL-6 stimulates osteoclast-like multinucleated cell formation in long term human marrow cultures by inducing IL-1 release. J Immunol 144:4226–4230

Lowe C, Cornish J, Martin TJ, Reid IR (1991) Effects of leukemia inhibitory factor on bone resorption and DNA synthesis in neonatal mouse calvaria. Calcif Tissue Int 49:394–397

MacDonald BR, Mundy GR, Wang EA, Kuehl TJ, Stanley ER, Roodman GD (1986) Effects of recombinant CSF-GM and highly purified CSF-1 on the formation of multinucleated cells with osteoclast characteristics in long-term bone marrow cultures. J Bone Miner Res 1:227–233

Martin TJ, Allan EH, Caple IW, Care AD, Danks JA, Diefenbach-Jagger H et al. (1989) Parathyroid hormone-related protein: isolation, molecular cloning, and mechanisms of action. Recent Prog Horm Res 45:467–506

Matsuda CL, Yamamoto N, Kaneko T, Iwahashi M, Hashimoto S, Araki K (1990) Hypercalcemia and serum TNF-alpha in T-cell leukemia. Lancet 28:1032

McDonell GD, Dunstan GR, Evans RA, Carter JN, Hills E, Wong SYP, McNeil DR (1982) Quantitative bone histology in the hypercalcemia of malignant disease. J Clin Endocrinol Metab 55:1066–1072
Mochizuki H, Hakeda Y, Wakatsuki N, Usui N, Akashi S, Sato T, Tanaka K, Kumegawa (1992) Insulin-like growth factor-I supports formation and activation of osteoclasts. Endocrinology 131:1075–1080
Moseley JM, Kubota M, Diefenbach-Jagger H, Wettenhall REH, Kemp BE, Suva LJ, Rodda CP, Ebeling PR, Hudson PJ, Zajac JD, Martin TJ (1987) Parathyroid hormone-related protein purified from a human lung cancer cell line. Proc Natl Acad Sci USA 84:5048–5052
Mundy GR (1989) Calcium homeostasis: hypercalcemia and hypocalcemia. Dunitz, London, pp 28–50
Mundy GR, Bertolini DB (1986) Bone destruction and hypercalcemia in plasma cell myeloma. Semin Oncol 13:291–299
Mundy GR, Martin TJ (1982) The hypercalcemia of malignancy: pathogenesis and management. Metabolism 31:1247–1277
Mundy GR, Roodman D (1987) Osteoclast ontogeny and function. In: Peck WA (ed) Bone and mineral research, vol 5. Elsevier, Amsterdam, p 209
Mundy GR, Raisz LG, Cooper RA, Schechter GP, Salmon SE (1974) Evidence for the secretion of an osteoclast stimulating factor in myeloma. N Engl J Med 291:1041–1046
Nathan C, Sporn M (1991) Cytokines in context. J Cell Biol 113:981–986
Nussbaum SR, Gaz RD, Arnold A (1990) Hypercalcemia and ectopic secretion of parathyroid hormone by an ovarian carcinoma with rearrangement of the gene for parathyroid hormone. N Engl J Med 323:1324–1328
Orcel P, Feuga M, Bielakoff J, de Vernejoul MC (1993) Local bone injections of LPS and M-CSF increase bone resorption by different pathways in vivo in rats. Am J Physiol 264:E391–E397
Ordffo ROC, Bonewald L, Kukita A, Garrett IR, Seyedin SM, Rosen D, Mundy GR (1990) Inhibitory effects of the bone-derived growth factors osteoinductive factor and transforming growth factor-β on isolated osteoclasts. Endocrinology 126:3069–3075
Passeri G, Girasole G, Knutson S, Yang Y-C, Manolagas SC, Jilka RL (1992) Interleukin 11 (IL-11): a new cytokine with osteoclastogenic and bone resorptive properties and a critical role in PTH- and 1,25(OH)2D_3-induced osteoclast development. J Bone Miner Res 8[Suppl 1]:S110
Pfeilschifter J, Seyedin SM, Mundy GR (1988) Transforming growth factor β inhibits bone resorption in fetal rat long bone cultures. J Clin Invest 82:680–685
Pfeilschifter J, Chenu C, Bird A, Mundy GR, Roodman GD (1989) Interleukin 1 and tumor necrosis factor stimulate the formation of human osteoclast-like cells in vitro. J Bone Miner Res 4:113–118
Pfeilschifter J, Bonewald L, Mundy GR (1990) Role of growth factors in cartilage and bone metabolism. In: Sporn MB, Roberts AB (eds) Peptide growth factors and their receptors II Springer, Berlin Heidelberg New York, pp 371–400
Pizurki L, Rizzoli R, Moseley J, Martin TJ, Caverzasio J, Bonjour J-P (1988) Effect of synthetic tumoral PTH-related peptide on cAMP production and Na-dependent Pi transport. Am J Physiol 255:F957–F961
Raisz LG, Simmons HA, Sandberg AL, Canalis E (1980) Direct stimulation of bone resorption by epidermal growth factor. Endocrinology 107:270–273
Ralston SH, Cowan RA, Robertson AG, Gardner MD, Boyle IT (1984) Circulating vitamin D metabolites and hypercalcemia of malignancy. Acta Endocrinol (Copenh) 106:556–563

Reid IR, Lowe C, Cornish J, Skinner SJM, Hilton DJ, Willson TA, Gearing DP, Martin TJ (1990) Leukemia inhibitory factor: a novel bone-active cytokine. Endocrinology 126:1416–1420
Rodan GA, Martin TJ (1981) Role of osteoblasts in hormonal control of bone resorption – a hypothesis. Calcif Tissue Int 33:349–351
Rosenthal N, Insogna KL, Godsall JW, Smaldone L, Waldron JA, Steward AF (1985) Elevations in circulating 1,25 dihydroxyvitamin D in three patients with lymphoma-associated hypercalcemia. J Clin Endocrinol Metab 60:29–33
Rosol TJ, Nagode LA, Couto CG, Hammer AS, Chew DJ, Peterson JL, Ayl RD, Steinmeyer CL, Capen CC (1992) Parathyroid hormone-related protein, parathyroid hormone, and 1,25-dihydroxyvitamin D in dogs with cancer-associated hypercalcemia. Endocrinology 131:1157–1164
Sabatini M, Boyce B, Aufdemorte T, Bonewald L, Mundy GR (1988) Infusions of recombinant human interleukins 1 alpha and 1 beta cause hypercalcemia in normal mice. Proc Natl Acad Sci USA 85:5235–5239
Salomon DS, Zweibel JA, Bano M et al. (1984) Presence of transforming growth factors in human breast cancer cells. Cancer Res 44:4069–4077
Sartori L, Weir EC, Steward AF, Broadus AE, Mangin M, Barrett P, Insogna KL (1988) Synthetic and partially-purified adenylate cyclase-stimulating proteins from tumors associated with humoral hypercalcemia of malignancy inhibit phosphate transport in a PTH-responsive renal cell line. J Clin Endocrinol Metab 66:459–461
Sato K, Fujii Y, Kasono K, Furutani Y, Yamada M, Shizume K (1987) Interleukin-1α and PTH-like factor are responsible for humoral hypercalcemia associated with esophageal carcinoma cells (EC-GI). J Bone Miner Res 2[Suppl 1]:387
Sato K, Fujii Y, Kasono K, Ozawa M, Imamura H, Kanaji Y, Kurosawa H, Tsushima T, Shizume K (1989) Parathyroid hormone-related protein and interleukin-1α synergistically stimulate bone resorption in vitro and increase the serum calcium concentration in mice in vivo. Endocrinology 124:2172–2178
Scheinmann SJ, Kelberman MW, Tatum AH, Zamkoff KW (1991) Case report: hypercalcemia with excess serum 1,25 dihydroxyvitamin D in lymphomatoid granulomatous/angiocentric lymphoma. Am J Med Sci 301:178–181
Shen V, Kohler G, Huang J, Huang SS, Peck WA (1989) An acidic fibroblast growth factor stimulates DNA synthesis, inhibits collagen and alkaline phosphatase synthesis and induces resorption in bone. Bone Miner 7:205–219
Shioi A, Teitelbaum SL, Ross FP, Welgus HG, Suzuki H, Ohara J, Lacey DL (1991) Interleukin 4 inhibits murine osteoclast formation in vitro. J Cell Biochem 47: 272–277
Simmons HA, Raisz LG (1991) Effects of acid and basic fibroblast growth factor and heparin on cultured fetal rat long bones. J Bone Miner Res 6:1301–1305
Slootweg MC, Most WW, van Beek E, Schot LPC, Papapoulos SE, Löwik CWGM (1992) Osteoclast formation together with interleukin-6 production in mouse long bones is increased by insulin-like growth factor-I. J Endocrinol 132:433–438
Sporn MB, Roberts AB (1988) Peptide growth factors are multifunctional. Nature 332:217–219
Sporn MB, Roberts AB (1990) (eds) Peptide growth factors and their receptors. Springer, Berlin Heidelberg New York
Steward AF, Horst R, Deftos LJ, Cadman EC, Lang R, Broadus AE (1980) Biochemical evaluation of patients with cancer-associated hypercalcemia evidence for humoral and nonhumoral groups. N Engl J Med 303:1377–1383
Steward AF, Vignery A, Silvergnte Ravin ND, Li Valsi V, Broadus AE, Baron R (1982) Quantitative bone histomorphometry in humoral hypercalcemia of malignancy: uncoupling of bone cell activity. J Clin Endocrinol Metab 55:219–227

Steward AF, Mangin M, Wu T, Goumas D, Insogna KL, Burtis WJ, Broadus AE (1988) Synthetic human parathyroid hormone-like protein stimulates bone resorption and causes hypercalcemia in rats. J Clin Invest 81:596–600

Steward AF, Elliot J, Burtis WJ, Wu T, Insogna KL (1989) Synthetic parathyroid hormone-like protein (1–74): biochemical and physiological characterization. Endocrinology 124:642–648

Suva LJ, Winslow GA, Wettenhall REH, Hammonds RG, Moseley JM, Diefenbach-Jagger H, Rodda CP, Kemp BE, Rodriguez H, Chen EY, Hudson PJ, Martin TJ, Wood WI (1987) A parathyroid hormone-related protein implicated in malignant hypercalcemia: cloning and expression. Science 237:893–896

Takahashi N, MacDonald BR, Hon J, Winkler ME, Derynck R, Mundy GR, Roodman GD (1986) Recombinant human transforming growth factor-alpha stimulates the formation of osteoclast-like cells in long-term human marrow cultures. J Clin Invest 78:894–898

Takahashi N, Udagawa N, Akatsu T, Tanaka H, Shionome M, Suda T (1991) Role of colony-stimulating factors in osteoclast development. J Bone Miner Res 6: 977–985

Tanaka S, Takahashi N, Udagawa N, Tamura T, Akatsu T, Stanley ER, Kurokawa T, Suda T (1993) Macrophage colony-stimulating factor is indispensable for both proliferation and differentiation of osteoclast progenitors. J Clin Invest 91: 257–263

Tashjian AH, Levine L (1978) Epidermal growth factor stimulates prostaglandin and bone resorption in cultured mouse calvaria. Biochem Biophys Res Commun 85:966–975

Tashjian AH, Hohmann EL, Antoniades HN, Levine L (1982) Platelet-derived growth factor stimulates bone resorption via a prostaglandin-mediated mechanism. Endocrinology 111:118–124

Tashjian AH, Voelkel EF, Lazzaro M, Singer FR, Roberts AB, Derynck R, Winkler ME, Levine L (1985) Alpha and beta transforming growth factors stimulate prostaglandin production and bone resorption in cultured mouse calvaria. Proc Natl Acad Sci USA 82:4535–4538

Tashjian AH, Voelkel EF, Lloyd W, Derynck R, Winkler ME, Levine L (1986) Actions of growth factors on plasma calcium: epidermal growth factor and human transforming growth factor-alpha cause elevation of plasma calcium in mice. J Clin Invest 78:1405–1409

Tashjian AH, Voelkel EF, Lazzaro M, Goad D, Bosma T, Levine L (1987) Tumor necrosis factor-alpha (cachectin) stimulates bone resorption in mouse calvaria via a prostaglandin-mediated mechanism. Endocrinology 120:2029–2036

Thomson BM, Saklatvala J, Chambers TJ (1986) Osteoblasts mediate interleukin 1 stimulation of bone resorption by rat osteoclasts. J Exp Med 164:104–112.

Thomson BM, Mundy GR, Chambers TJ (1987) Tumor mecrosis factors alpha and beta induce osteoblastic cells to stimulate osteoclastic bone resorption. J Immunol 138:775–779

Thorikay M, Kramer S, Reynolds F, Sorvillo JM, Doescher L, Morris CA, Burtis WJ, Insogna KL, Valenzuela DM, Steward AF (1989) Synthesis of a gene encoding parathyroid hormone-like protein (1–141): purification and biological characterization of the expressed protein. Endocrinology 124:111–118

Watanabe K, Tanaka Y, Morimoto I, Yahata K, Zeki K, Fujihira T, Yamashita U, Eto S (1990) Interleukin-4 as a potent inhibitor of bone resorption. Biochem Biophys Res Commun 172:1035–1041

Wiktor-Jedzrejczak W, Bartocci A, Ferrante AW, Ahmed-Ansari A, Sell KW, Pollard JW, Stanley ER (1990) Total absence of colony-stimulating factor 1 in the macrophage-deficient osteopetrotic (op/op) mouse. Proc Natl Acad Sci USA 87:4828–4832

Yamamoto I, Kitamura N, Aoki J, Kawamura J, Dokoh S, Morita R, Torizuka K (1987) Circulating 1,25-dihydroxyvitamin D concentrations in patients with renal cell carcinoma-associated hypercalcemia are rarely suppressed. J Clin Endocrinol Metab 64:175–179

Yates AJP, Gutierrez GE, Smolens P, Travis PS, Katz MS, Aufdemorte TB, Boyce BF, Hymer TK, Poser JW, Mundy GR (1988) Effects of a synthetic peptide of a parathyroid hormone-related protein on calcium homeostasis, renal tubular calcium reabsorption, and bone metabolism in vivo and in vitro in rodents. J Clin Invest 81:932–938

Yates AJ, Boyce BF, Favarato G, Aufdemorte TB, Marcelli C, Kester MB, Walker R, Langton BC, Bonewald LF, Mundy GR (1992) Expression of human transforming growth factor alpha by Chinese hamster ovarian tumors in nude mice causes hypercalcemia and increased osteoclastic bone resorption. J Bone Miner Res 7:847–853

Yoneda T, Alsina MM, Chavez JB, Bonewald L, Mundy GR (1989) Hypercalcemia in a human tumor is due to tumor mecrosis factor production by host immune cells. J Bone Miner Res 4:826

Yoshida H, Hayashi S-I, Kunisada T, Ogawa M, Nishikawa S, Okamura H, Sudo T, Shultz LD, Nishikawa S-I (1990) The murine mutation osteopetrosis in the coding region of the macrophage colony stimulating factor gene. Nature 345:442–446

Yoshimoto K, Yamasaki R, Sakai H, Tezuka U, Takahashi M, Tizuka M, Sekiya T, Saito S (1989) Ectopic production of parathyroid hormone by small cell lung cancer in a patient with hypercalcemia. J Clin Endocrinol Metab 68:976–981

Humoral Hypercalcemia of Malignancy: Role of Parathyroid Hormone-Related Protein

E. Blind

Department of Internal Medicine I – Endocrinology and Metabolism, University of Heidelberg, Bergheimerstraße 58, 69115 Heidelberg, Germany

Introduction: Discovery of Parathyroid Hormone-Related Protein (PTHrP)

Hypercalcemia is a frequent complication of many types of malignancy (Mundy 1985). The humoral form of the syndrome (humoral hypercalcemia of malignancy, HHM) causes hypercalcemia without necessarily metastasizing to the bone and shares several biochemical features with primary hyperparathyroidism (pHPT), such as hypercalcemia and hypophosphatemia in plasma, and decreased renal reabsorption of phosphorus. An excess of parathyroid hormone (PTH) is, of course, the cause of hypercalcemia in pHPT, leading F. Albright more than half a century ago to the suggestion that PTH or a PTH-like factor might be involved in HHM. In the 1970s, with the availability of PTH immunoassays, it became evident that PTH itself usually was not the factor responsible for HHM.

Several clinical studies pointed to a PTH-like factor in HHM, such as the study performed by A.F. Stewart et al. in 1980: They were able to demonstrate similarly elevated levels of urinary cAMP in 80% of patients with hypercalcemia of malignancy (Fig. 1), thus showing that a substance interacting with the renal PTH receptor was involved. Urinary cAMP is usually elevated in pHPT and is thought to be a highly specific marker for the action of PTH on renal PTH receptors, whereby the stimulation of adenylate cyclase in renal tubular cells leads to increased urinary cAMP. Therefore, the detection of this factor became possible by the use of in vitro bioassays, most of them based on the stimulation of adenylate cyclase via the PTH/PTHrP receptor in bone or kidney cells. This led to the simultaneous isolation and purification of parathyroid hormone-related protein (PTHrP) from human breast, lung, and renal carcinomas (Burtis et al. 1987; Moseley et al. 1987; Strewler et al. 1987) and the subsequent cloning of the cDNA (Mangin et al. 1988a; Suva et al. 1987; Thiede et al. 1988). PTHrP mRNA isolated from several tissues encoded PTHrPs of different lengths, between 139 and 173 amino acids, with an identical common sequence (Burtis et al.

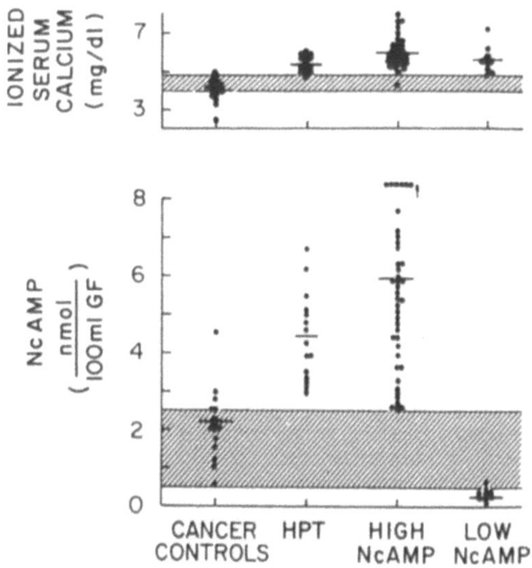

Fig. 1. Nephrogenous cyclic AMP (NcAMP) and ionized serum calcium in four patient groups (*from left to right*): 15 normocalcemic cancer patients, 15 patients with primary hyperparathyroidism (*HPT*), 41 patients with hypercalcemia of malignancy and elevated NcAMP (*HHM*; mostly squamous carcinomas, renal carcinomas, and carcinomas of the bladder) and 9 with suppressed NcAMP (local osteolytic form; mostly breast carcinomas and hematologic malignancies). *Hatched areas* represent the normal range. (From Stewart et al. 1980)

1987; Mangin et al. 1988b; Thiede et al. 1988). The PTHrP gene (on chromosome 12) is more complex than the gene for PTH (on chromosome 11), both of which are apparently derived from the same ancestor gene during evolution. The gene consists of nine exons, different promoters, and generates multiple mRNA transcripts by alternative splicing (Mangin et al. 1989, 1990; Suva et al. 1989; Yasuda et al. 1989).

The N-terminal ends of PTHrP and PTH have eight identical amino acid residues (Fig. 2) and have very similar biological activities on bone and kidney. The amino acid sequence is highly conserved between species through amino acid 111 (Fig. 2), but the actual circulating forms are not known.

Effect of PTHrP on Bone and Kidney In Vitro and In Vivo

Humoral hypercalcemia of malignancy shares several biochemical features with pHPT, closely reflecting the similarities of PTH an PTHrP action on bone and kidney. PTH an PTHrP interact with similar affinities to identical receptors on osteoblast-like cells (Jüppner et al. 1988; Nissenson et al. 1988) and with receptors on canine renal membranes (Orloff et al. 1989). This is at

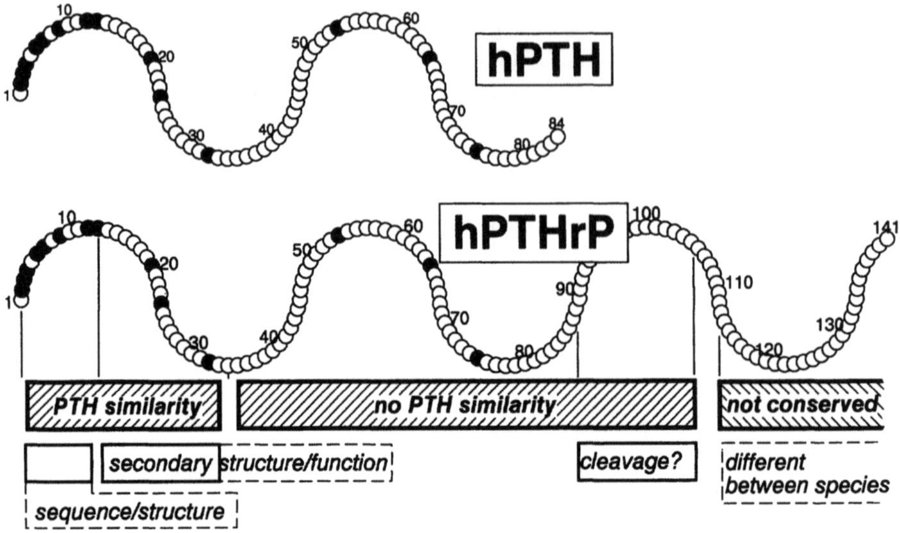

Fig. 2. Features of parathyroid hormone-related protein. Shown is the human sequence PTHrP (1–141). Amino acids identical with human parathyroid hormone PTH (1–84) are represented by *closed circles*

least in part due to the sequence homology of the peptides at their N-terminal ends, 8 out of the first 13 amino acids being identical (Fig. 2). The N-terminal fragment 1–34 of both PTH an PTHrP is able to elicit most classic effects on target cells of calcium homeostasis in almost equipotent doses (Fig. 3). The C-terminal part beyond amino acid residue 13 is required for this (presumably to bind to the receptor). Surprisingly, the sequence of both peptides is completely different in this stretch (Fig. 2), and one must assume a high degree of similarity in secondary structure. A number of in vitro studies have shown nearly identical effects with similar doses of N-terminal fragments (usually the sequence 1–34) of PTH and PTHrP on bone cells, such as: stimulation of adenylate cyclase, a hallmark of the effect of this peptide on osteoblast metabolism (Blind et al. 1993a; Horiochu et al. 1987; Kemp et al. 1987; Stewart et al. 1988), inhibition of alkaline phosphatase and growth of osteoblast-like cells (Rodan et al. 1988), and, although somewhat differing effects between both peptides have been described, activation of the intracellular calcium second messenger system (Civitelli et al. 1989; Yamada et al. 1989). Identical cDNAs for a PTH/PTHrP receptor have been cloned recently from human bone and kidney (Schipani et al. 1993), and identical cDNAs have also been found in rat bone (Abou-Samra et al. 1992) versus kidney cells. Therefore, although unique PTHrP receptors may well exist (see below), there is to date no strong evidence that PTHrP would act on classic organs of calcium homeostasis (bone and kidney) other than via the shared PTH/PTHrP receptor.

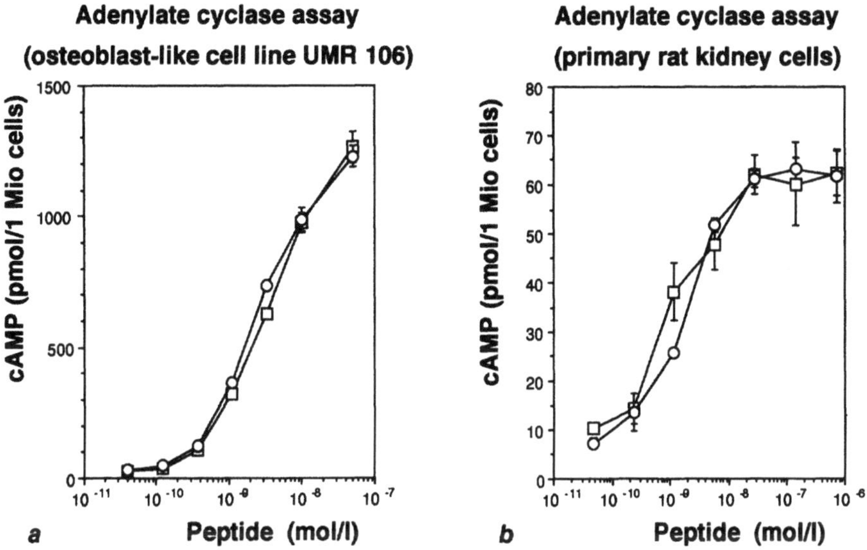

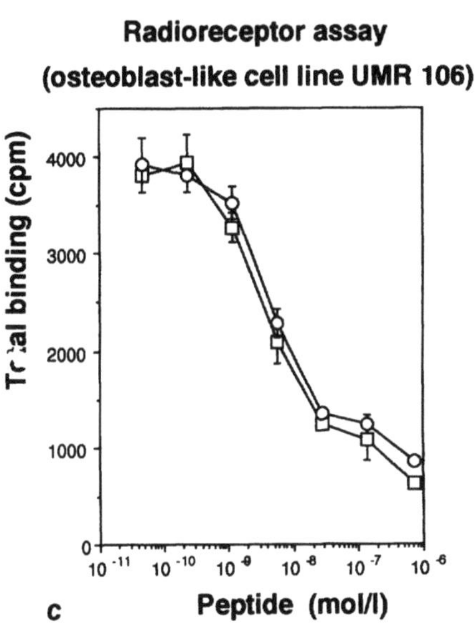

Fig. 3a–c. PTH/PTHrP-stimulated cAMP accumulation and PTH/PTHrP binding in rat bone and kidney cells: rat kidney cells from primary culture (**a**) and clonal rat osteoblast-like cells (UMR 106) (**b**) after stimulation for 15 min by N-terminal rat PTH [rPTH (1–34); □] and N-terminal rat PTHrP [rPTHrP (1–34); ○]. Assays were performed as described (Blind et al. 1993a). Displacement of ^{125}I-labeled PTHrP (1–86) from the receptors of UMR 106 cells by the same N-terminal fragments of PTH/PTHrP (**c**)

Since animal models of hypercalcemia of malignancy are discussed elsewhere in this book (see chapter by T. Schilling), the evidence for PTHrP being the main factor in HHM is only briefly mentioned here: In several animal models, synthetic PTHrPs can cause all the hallmarks of PTH action, such as hypercalcemia, hyperphosphaturia, elevated nephrogenous cAMP, and stimulation of osteoclastic bone resorption. Exogenous N-terminal fragments of PTHrP act similarly to PTH in man (Fraher et al. 1992). Furthermore, infusion of antibodies against PTHrP is able to reverse hypercalcemia and other manifestations in experimental HHM. This shows clearly that PTHrP is the necessary (although may be not entirely sufficient) factor to cause HHM in these models.

Some discrepancies between the clinical pictures of HHM and pHPT with regard to bone and kidney still exist. Although PTH and PTHrP act similarly on osteoblast-like cells in vitro, bone formation seems to be relatively lower in HHM than in pHPT (Stewart et al. 1982), in the presence of increased bone resorption in both cases. Depressed bone formation in HHM might be caused by differences of action of PTHrP compared to PTH, but might as well result from release of additional substances, such as cytokines, from tumors, or might be more indirectly caused by less specific effects of severe malignant disease.

Another discrepancy is the level of 1,25-dihydroxyvitamin D_3 in circulation: 1,25-dihydroxyvitamin D_3 is often elevated in patients with pHPT, but tends to be low in HHM (Stewart et al. 1980). By contrast, animals after short-term infusion of PTHrP, as well as tumor-bearing animals in HHM models, have increased levels of 1,25-dihydroxyvitamin D_3. There are several possible explanations, among them the existence of a factor released by one tumor, which inhibits the renal 1-α-hydroxylase (Fukumoto et al. 1989). Data from our own group showed suppressed levels of 1,25-dihydroxyvitamin D_3 in HHM despite high PTHrP levels, which rebound, however, after calcium-lowering therapy. This suggested a more effective inhibition of the renal 1-α-hydroxylase by high serum calcium levels overcoming the possible stimulatory effect of PTHrP, among the other possibilities discussed in the paper (Schilling et al. 1993).

Measuring PTHrP in Plasma

There is now a growing number of published immunoassays for PTHrP, either site-specific radioimmunoassays (RIAs) or two-site assays. Since the known PTH-like biological activity of PTHrP is located within the first 34 amino acids, most of the first RIAs have been directed against the N-terminal sequence of PTHrP (Budayr et al. 1989b; Grill et al. 1991; Henderson et al. 1990; Kao et al. 1990; Ratcliffe and Ratcliffe 1990). Although N-terminal PTHrP has been measured in plasma by direct RIA (Grill et al. 1991; Henderson et al. 1990; Ratcliffe et al. 1991b; Scharla et al. 1991), prior extraction steps were often required to obtain clinically useful results (Budayr et al. 1989b; Kao et al. 1990). This situation resembled the difficulties with assays for N-terminal PTH and may be complicated by the very low levels (<2.5 pmol/l) of N-terminal PTHrP extracted by immunoaffinity chromatography from normal serum (Budayr et al. 1989b). More sensitive assays have been developed by applying the two-site immunoradiometric assay (IRMA) technique to detect PTHrP of the approximate amino acid sequences 1–74 to 1–86 (Burtis et al. 1990; Pandian et al. 1992; Ratcliffe et al. 1991a). The topic has been reviewed recently (Burtis 1992) (see also below and chapter by H. Schmidt-Gayk). These assays are now helpful in diagnosing HHM, but are still not yet sufficient to detect PTHrP in normal persons reliably.

PTHrP in Humoral Hypercalcemia of Malignancy

Several different studies have now shown the involvement of PTHrP in the pathogenesis of humoral hypercalcemia of malignancy (HHM) by demonstrating elevated plasma levels of PTHrP in the vast majority of patients suffering from the syndrome. An early RIA for N-terminal PTHrP (using immunoaffinity chromatography as a preceding extraction step) found elevated levels in 33 of 48 (69%) patients with a solid tumor and hypercalcemia (Budayr et al. 1989b). Another N-terminal RIA (Kao et al. 1990) detected 12 of 25 patients (48%).

Our group has developed an RIA for the midregional part of the protein, as described elsewhere (Blind et al. 1992). In brief, the assay cross-reacts with PTHrP (1–86) and PTHrP (53–84), and uses a goat antiserum against amino acid residues 53–84, synthetic human PTHrP (1–86) as a standard, and radiolabeled PTHrP (1–86) as tracer. The assay has a lower limit of detection of 5 pmol/l and the upper limit of the normal range is 21 pmol/l. With this assay, we studied a total of 94 patients with hypercalcemia of malignancy (the tumor types are summarized in Table 1, together with additional parameters). Intact PTH was measured simultaneously to exclude the patients with concomitant pHPT. Of 32 patients with pHPT, 30 had midregional PTHrP concentrations within the normal range and only two had slightly elevated levels (Fig. 4). Of 38 patients with a solid tumor and normocalcemia, only one had elevated midregional PTHrP concentrations, but remained normocalcemic so far (Fig. 4).

Among the 73 patients with solid tumors and hypercalcemia, 44 (60%) had elevated PTHrP levels (Fig. 4, Table 1). The concentrations ranged from undetectable (<5 pmol/l) to 333 pmol/l (median, 29 pmol/l). In these patients, serum total calcium was positively correlated with midregional PTHrP levels ($p = 0.018$). Intact PTH levels were either suppressed or within the normal range in all patients. The frequency of elevated PTHrP levels and tumor type is shown in Table 1. PTHrP was most often elevated (in 81%) in patients suffering from squamous type tumors (Table 1).

This RIA of midregional PTHrP provided high diagnostic sensitivity (60%) in the identification of patients with hypercalcemia associated with solid tumors, especially of the squamous type (81%). This is comparable with results of other assays against different sequences of PTHrP. The sensitive and specific two-site assay methodology may allow detection of

Table 1. Serum concentrations of PTHrP, PTH, and calcium in 94 patients with hypercalcemia of malignancy. (Reprinted in modified form from Blind et al. 1993c)

Type of Malignancy	*n*	Bone metastases (%)	PTHrP (pmol/l) Median (range)	PTHrP (% elev.)	S-calcium (mmol/l) Median (range)	Intact PTH (ng/l) Median
Solid						
Lung	12	17	48 (<5–95)	83	2.84 (2.73–3.40)	10
Breast	19	84	21 (<5–86)	53	3.12 (2.80–4.10)	8
Bladder	4	50	34 (<5–98)	50	2.83 (2.72–3.13)	29
Kidney	9	44	20 (7–333)	44	2.98 (2.70–3.78)	5
Liver	7	14	57 (16–203)	86	3.17 (2.76–3.80)	10
Esophagus	3	33	9 (<5–14)	0	3.53 (2.78–4.43)	16
Others/ squamous	11	36	29 (<5–141)	73	3.10 (2.80–5.02)	5
Others/non-squamous	8	13	24 (<5–63)	50	3.03 (2.72–3.96)	4
Total	73	42	29 (<5–333)	60	3.02 (2.70–5.02)	11
Of which:						
Squamous type	21	29	42 (<5–141)	81	2.97 (2.73–5.02)	
With bone metastases	31	100	21 (<5–141)	48	3.10 (2.80–4.10)	
Without bone metastases	35	0	31 (<5–333)	66	2.98 (2.70–5.02)	
Hematologic						
Plasmocytoma	4	–	13 (<5–30)	27	2.94 (2.73–3.86)	16
NHL	6	–	13 (8–20)	0	2.77 (2.70–3.55)	18
Others	11	–	13 (<5–20)	0	2.76 (2.72–2.81)	17
Total	21	–	13 (<5–30)	14	2.85 (2.70–3.86)	17

PTHrP was measured by RIA against midregional PTHrP (Blind et al. 1992) (normal range: <5–21 pmol/l). Intact PTH was determined by an immunochemoluminometric two-site assay (normal range: 10–65 ng/l; Ciba Corning, Fernwald, Germany). Total serum calcium was determined by flame photometry (normal range: 2.10–2.65 mmol/l).

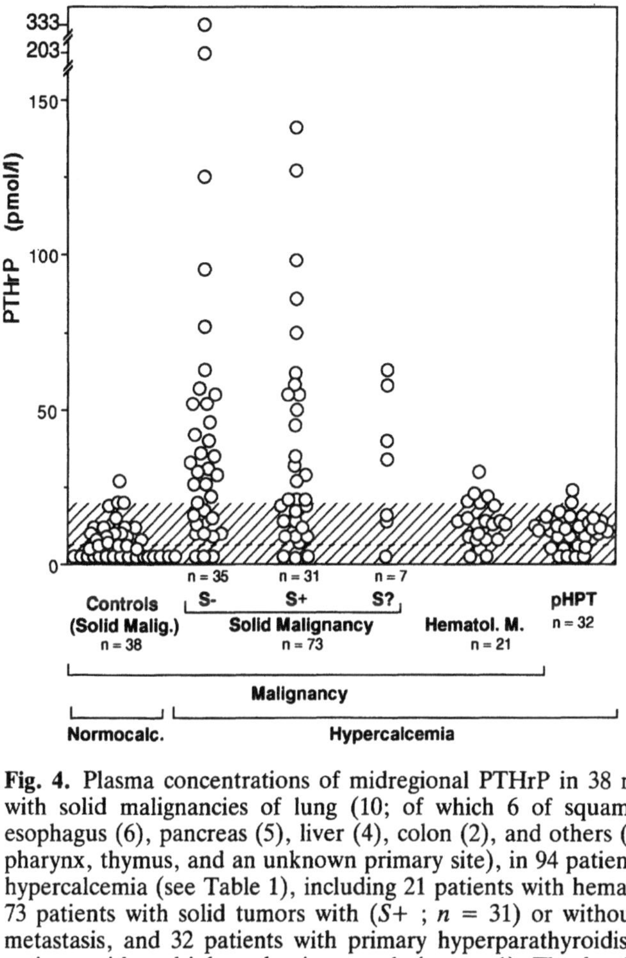

Fig. 4. Plasma concentrations of midregional PTHrP in 38 normocalcemic patients with solid malignancies of lung (10; of which 6 of squamous type), breast (6), esophagus (6), pancreas (5), liver (4), colon (2), and others (5; rectum, gallbladder, pharynx, thymus, and an unknown primary site), in 94 patients with malignancy and hypercalcemia (see Table 1), including 21 patients with hematologic malignancy and 73 patients with solid tumors with ($S+$; $n = 31$) or without ($S-$; $n = 35$) bone metastasis, and 32 patients with primary hyperparathyroidism (pHPT, including 3 patients with multiple endocrine neoplasia type 1). The *hatched area* represents the normal range of midregional PTHrP; the *hatched line* indicates the limit of detection (= 5 pmol/l). (Modified from Blind et al. 1993c)

PTHrP in even more cases. With the first PTHrP assay of that kind, PTHrP (1–74) was found to be elevated in approximately 80% of a similar group of patients (Burtis et al. 1990) (Fig. 5). Recently, elevated PTHrP (1–86) in 90%–95% of patients of a similar group has been reported (Pandian et al. 1992; Ratcliffe et al. 1991a).

In several studies PTHrP levels and calcium in plasma were positively correlated in HHM patients as were PTHrP levels and urinary cAMP concentrations (Burtis et al. 1990), which logically follows from the causal relationship between PTHrP secretion and hypercalcemia. Since PTHrP secretion by tumor tissue should precede the development of hypercalcemia, one could expect PTHrP elevations in still normocalcemic tumor patients.

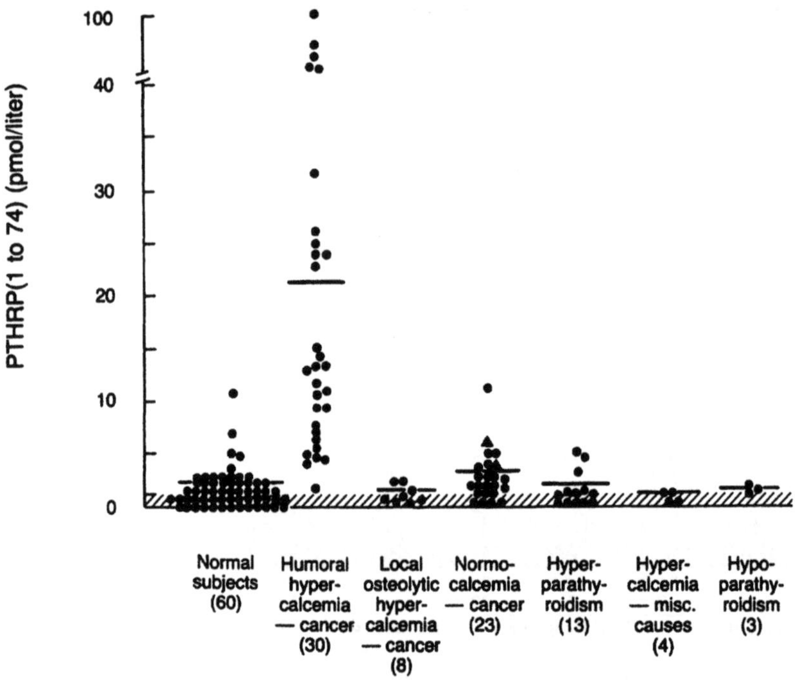

Fig. 5. Plasma concentrations of PTHrP (1–74) as measured by two-site assay in 60 normal subjects and in 61 patients with malignancy. Also shown are patients with hyperparathyroidism, hypoparathyroidism, and hypercalcemia due to other causes. The *hatched area* represents undetectable PTHrP levels, ▲ indicates two normocalcemic patients with cancer who subsequently became hypercalcemic. (From Burtis et al. 1990)

This is in fact the case in a small percentage of normocalcemic tumor patients (Bundred et al. 1991; Burtis et al. 1990), a percentage that might rise with even more sensitive assays yet to come. Measuring PTHrP in normocalcemic patients may then have prognostic relevance (Heath 1993).

PTHrP in Local Osteolytic Hypercalcemia of Solid Malignancies

For a long time, it was assumed that in patients with radiologic evidence of extensive skeletal destruction by malignancy (especially in breast cancer), local osteolytic hypercalcemia (LOH) was the mechanism responsible. However, the severity of hypercalcemia and the extent of bone metastasis was often not closely correlated. Several studies challenged the importance of metastasis alone for hypercalcemia by finding elevated levels of PTHrP with similar frequency in patients with bone metastasis compared with patients without bone metastasis, such as our study (Fig. 4, Table 1, 48% vs.

66%): Median PTHrP levels were only slightly higher in patients without bone involvement (median: 31 vs. 21 pmol/l), but this difference was not statistically significant. Our 31 patients with metastatic skeletal disease had only slightly higher serum calcium concentrations than our 35 patients with no evidence of bone involvement (median: 3.10 vs. 2.98 mmol/l; Fig. 4, Table 1). In fact, the local osteolytic form is indistinguishable from the humoral form solely by the presence or absence of skeletal metastasis (Bilezikian 1990, 1991), since our and other's studies (Burtis et al. 1990; Grill et al. 1991; Henderson et al. 1990; Kao et al. 1990) have demonstrated HHM in the presence and absence of bone involvement. Instead, the diagnosis of HHM relies largely on the demonstration of elevated plasma PTHrP levels or elevated urinary excretion of cyclic AMP, as another independent marker (Stewart et al. 1980), both of which were strongly correlated in this syndrome (Burtis et al. 1990).

Especially remarkable are the results in patients with breast cancer: 10 out of our 19 patients had elevated PTHrP levels, in the presence of bone metastasis in almost all patients (Table 1). This result was almost identical with the experience of the Australian group, where 13 patients had elevated PTHrP out of 20 similar patients (Grill et al. 1991). Another recent study found elevated PTHrP in 92% of patients with breast cancer, hypercalcemia, and bone metastasis, and in 36% of normocalcemic patients with bone metastasis (Bundred et al. 1991) Fifty to 60% of breast cancer tissue is immunocytochemically positive for PTHrP (Bundred et al. 1991; Southby et al. 1990), but 92% of metastasis in bone has found to be PTHrP-positive compared to 17% of metastasis in other sites (Powell et al. 1991). Therefore, it has been suggested that PTHrP-positive tumors might be more likely to metastasize to bone, possibly due to local action of PTHrP. This would imply possible therapeutic consequences, since such a subgroup of patients may be treated prophylactically with bisphosphonates (Heath 1993).

Humoral Mechanisms in Hematologic Malignancies

The mechanism of hypercalcemia is apparently very different in hematologic malignancies. The majority of our patients with hematologic malignancies had normal midregional PTHrP levels (Fig. 4, Table 1). Two patients with multipe myeloma had slightly elevated PTHrP levels (22 and 23 pmol/l), and in only one patient was PTHrP clearly elevated (30 pmol/l). This is in agreement with most other results, such as the study by Budayr et al. (1989b), who found elevated N-terminal PTHrP in only 3 of 14 patients, although some early reports found higher percentages of elevated PTHrP in small numbers of patients (Henderson et al. 1990; Kao et al. 1990).

Thus, PTHrP seems to be of little pathogenetic importance in hematologic malignancies, with the two exceptions of adult T-cell leukemia/lymphoma (Fukumoto et al. 1988; Motokura et al. 1988) and possibly some plasmocytomas. The underlying mechanisms of nonhumoral hypercalcemia in hematologic malignancies are discussed elsewhere (see chapter by A. Grauer).

Circulating Forms of PTHrP

Circulating forms of PTHrP, especially those not containing the amino terminus, have been characterized very insufficiently by immunoassays so far (Soifer and Stewart 1992). Our immunoassay was directed against PTHrP residues 53–84 (Blind et al. 1992), a sequence chosen because this epitope was distinct from the region associated with PTH-like bioactivity and was likely to be contained in most circulating forms of PTHrP, based on reports of the molecular size of PTHrP in plasma and in tumor extracts (Burtis et al. 1987; Henderson et al. 1990; Moseley et al. 1987).

Midregional PTHrP levels as measured by our assay were about tenfold higher than N-terminal PTHrP levels (upper limit of normal: <2 pmol/l (Grill et al. 1991); 2.5 pmol/l (Budayr et al. 1989b); 5 pmol/l (Kao et al. 1990)), probably because our assay detects PTHrP fragments which do not cross-react in N-terminal assays of PTHrP. The assay detected PTHrP (1–86) by recognizing epitopes within the sequence 53–84. Immunoassayable PTHrP (56–86) was found to circulate in levels up to 35 ng/1 (Mitlak et al. 1991), and another RIA, against PTHrP (37–67), detected much higher mean concentrations of 320 pmol/l PTHrP in normals (Ratcliffe et al. 1991b), despite the fact that the antiserum used in this assay compared with our antiserum was thought to recognize a nearby epitope spanning residues 52–61 (Ratcliffe et al. 1991b). This assay, however, showed poor discrimination between normals and patients with humoral hypercalcemia of malignancy. PTHrP measured with an RIA against PTHrP (109–138) (Burtis et al. 1990) was also very different from PTHrP detected with our assay, since PTHrP (109–138) increased to a large degree in renal failure. Further characterization of circulating peptides showed at least two fractions, one of an M_r of approximately 6500 representing presumably the first 50–60 amino acid residues and a larger C-terminal fragment of an M_r of approximately 12 000 (Burtis et al. 1992). Our own results with a direct comparison of midregional PTHrP levels and levels measured with a commercially available two-site IRMA detecting PTHrP (1–72) (Nichols Institute) (Blind et al. 1993b) also showed heterogeneity of circulating forms (Fig. 6): Median midregional PTHrP was 34 pmol/l, which was about tenfold higher than the median of the PTHrP IRMA values (2.2 pmol/l). Furthermore, although PTHrP levels obtained with these two assays were significantly correlated, some patients had only elevated levels in one assay, suggesting different secretion patterns of individual tumors.

There is increasing evidence that PTHrP undergoes extensive post-translational processing, including probably cleavage and glycosylation (Wu

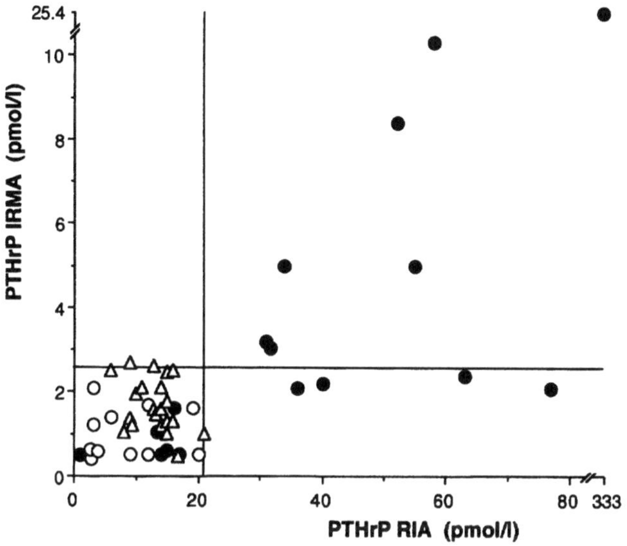

Fig. 6. Evidence of immunoheterogeneity of circulating PTHrP by measurement by RIA for the midregional sequence of PTHrP (*x*-axis) and by two-site IRMA (*y*-axis; Nichols). Concentrations of PTHrP in serum or plasma of 17 patients with hypercalcemia of malignancy (●) (serum calcium: 3.05 ± 0.36 mmol/l, mean ± SD, 16 solid tumors of the lung (5), breast (3), and kidney (2), one with non-Hodgkin's lymphoma), 11 normocalcemic patients with malignancy (○) (10 of them with lung carcinoma), and 21 control subjects. (From Blind et al. 1993b)

et al. 1991). In principle, cleavage can occur in circulation, but recent results also show intracellular endoproteolytic cleavage prior to secretion (de Papp et al. 1993). This complex situation easily explains different results with individual immunoassays. Furthermore, secreted forms of PTHrP might well be tissue specific and might even have different targets, as suggested in the paragraph about physiologic functions of PTHrP (see below).

Effect of Therapy on PTHrP Secretion and Action

Very little is known about the regulation of PTHrP secretion. Some in vitro studies showed inhibition of PTHrP release by chromogranin A and stimulation by calcitonin in a human lung tumor cell line (BEN) (Deftos et al. 1989). In other studies, PTHrP mRNA levels in the human cell line TT (Ikeda et al. 1989) and PTHrP in the supernatant of Walker 256 carcinosarcoma cells (Wagner et al. 1993) were lowered by dexamethasone and 1,25-dihydroxyvitamin D_3.

Leydig tumor cells, which are derived from an animal model of humoral hypercalcemia of malignancy, produced more PTHrP in the presence of elevated extracellular calcium, comparable to the concentration in vivo (Rizzoli and Bonjour 1989). Therefore, it has been hypothesized that increases in serum calcium in patients with HHM might increase the secretion rate of PTHrP by these tumors, thus aggravating hypercalcemia. To test this hypothesis, we recently examined calcium regulation and its effects on the release of PTHrP by tumors during rapid decrease of serum calcium in HHM patients by bisphosphonates (Blind et al. 1993d). The biochemical profiles of our patients are shown in Table 2. After a single infusion of the bisphosphonate, serum calcium concentrations decreased in all patients, with a maximal effect after 4–6 days (an example is shown in Fig. 7). In the group with elevated PTHrP, the calcium-lowering effect of the drug was significantly less pronounced than in the group with normal PTHrP levels (2.89 vs. 2.51 mmol/l serum calcium at day 6, Table 2), despite similar calcium values at the beginning. At day 6 after administration of the drug, five out of six patients with elevated PTHrP were still hypercalcemic, whereas only one out of four patients with normal PTHrP remained hypercalcemic. In both groups of patients, PTHrP levels remained unchanged 6 days after administration of the calcium-lowering drug as compared with pretherapeutic values (Table 2). Apparently, neither the drug itself nor the rapid fall in serum calcium seemed to influence the release of PTHrP by the tumors.

The calcium-lowering effect of the bisphosphonate BM 21.0955 was less effective in patients with elevated PTHrP than in patients with normal levels. This compares well with results with pamidronate, where the number of days to achieve normocalcemia was positively correlated with PTHrP levels before therapy (Dodwell et al. 1991). PTHrP levels might therefore predict the effectiveness of bisphosphonate therapy.

Beyond that, these results point to the underlying mechanism of hypercalcemia mediated by PTHrP. Before assays for PTHrP became widely available, it had been postulated that bisphosphonates were less effective in HHM compared with LOH (Gurney et al. 1989). In addition, the response to inhibitors of bone resorption remained incomplete when calcium reabsorption by the kidney was elevated due to a humorally mediated mechanism (Ralston et al. 1985, 1987). The renal contribution to hypercalcemia in this setting is mediated by PTHrP. Both findings were confirmed directly by administration of a bisphosphonate to rats perfused with PTHrP (Rizzoli et al. 1989). The weaker response of patients with high PTHrP to bisphosphonates may therefore be attributable to the effect of PTHrP-mediated renal calcium reabsorption on hypercalcemia in these patients, an effect which is not influenced by bisphosphonates. Additionally, high PTHrP levels might result in a more powerful stimulation of bone resorption, requiring higher doses of bisphosphonates (Dodwell et al. 1991).

Reduction of tumor mass by surgery or chemotherapy has been shown to lower circulating levels of PTHrP and subsequently serum calcium levels. Surgery, however, is rarely performed in advanced cases of HHM. As an

Table 2. Effect of therapy with the bisphosphonate BM 21.0955 on serum PTHrP, PTH, calcium, and creatinine levels in serum of ten patients with hypercalcemia of malignancy. (Reprinted from Blind et al. 1993d)

Parameter	Normal range	Day	Patients with normal PTHrP ($n = 4$)[a]	Patients with elevated PTHrP ($n = 6$)[b]	All patients ($n = 10$)
Midregional PTHrP	<5–21 pmol/l	0	17.8 ± 3.4	58.2 ± 37.3	42.0 ± 34.8
		6	15.0 ± 8.3[c]	60.0 ± 35.4[c]	42.0 ± 35.5[c]
Intact PTH	10–65 ng/l	0	15.7 ± 4.8	11.8 ± 3.8	13.4 ± 4.4
		6	19.7 ± 13.7	17.0.± 9.5	18.1 ± 10.7
Corrected serum calcium	2.10–2.65 mmol/l	0	3.43 ± 0.56	3.44 ± 0.37	3.42 ± 0.42
		6	2.51 ± 0.07[d]	2.89 ± 0.27[d]	2.74 ± 0.29
Serum creatinine	<1.3 mg/100 ml	0	0.95 ± 0.34	1.42 ± 0.74	1.23 ± 0.63
		6	0.85 ± 0.25	1.18 ± 0.41	1.05 ± 0.83

The bisphosphonate was administered as a single dose of 0.2–1.6 mg over 4 h intravenously. Values are means ± SD. Determinations at 0 and 6 days after treatment.

[a] Patients had rhabdomyosarcoma, pancreatic carcinoma, multiple myeloma, and non-Hodgkin's lymphoma, with bone metastases in one case and PTHrP concentrations from 15 to 21 pmol/l.

[b] Patients had carcinoma of the breast (two), lung, bladder, liver, and tumor of an unknown primary site (squamous carcinoma), with bone metastases in four cases and PTHrP concentrations from 25 to 118 pmol/l.

[c] Not significantly different from concentration before therapy ($p < 0.05$).

[d] Different between patients with normal and raised PTHrP ($p < 0.05$).

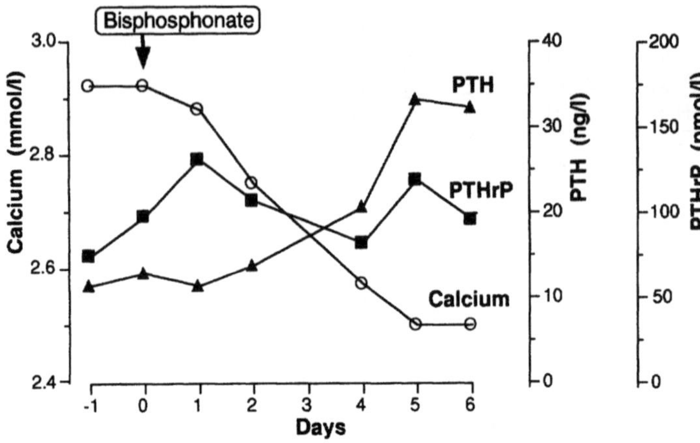

Fig. 7. Typical PTH and PTHrP plasma levels in HHM during calcium-lowering therapy: concentrations of serum calcium (○), intact PTH (▲), and midregional PTHrP (■) in a patient with hypercalcemia of malignancy and elevated levels of PTHrP before and after a single intravenous dose of 0.6 mg of the bisphosphonate BM 21.0955. (From Blind et al. 1993d)

example of the effect of chemotherapy, we present a patient who received chemotherapy with several cycles of etoposide (Vepesid) together with a calcium-lowering therapy with different bisphosphonates administered i.v. over 3 months (Fig. 8). Again, the bisphophonate alone was able to lower serum calcium but had no sustained influence on the PTHrP levels. Additional chemotherapy, however, resulted in a substantial decline in PTHrP levels, accompanied by a fall in serum calcium (Fig. 8).

Other Mediators of HHM: Role of Parathyroid Hormone

In the 1970s, a number of factors were considered to be mediators of HHM, among them PTH and PTH precursors, vitamin D metabolites, and other substances such as prostaglandins.

In some studies, early immunoassays for PTH showed elevated levels in a percentage (although often small) of patients with hypercalcemia and malignancy. But in the late 1980s, highly specific and sensitive two-site assays for PTH became available, showing uniformly suppressed or low normal levels of PTH in HHM (and in any other nonparathyroid hypercalcemia) (Blind et al. 1988). These new two-site PTH assays improved the differential diagnosis of hypercalcemia substantially (see chapter by H. Schmidt-Gayk), and it became clear that ectopic production of PTH by nonparathyroid tumors (also called true pseudohyperparathyroidism) is extremely rare. This was in accordance with the failure to detect PTH mRNA in a small number of nonparathyroid tumors associated with hyper-

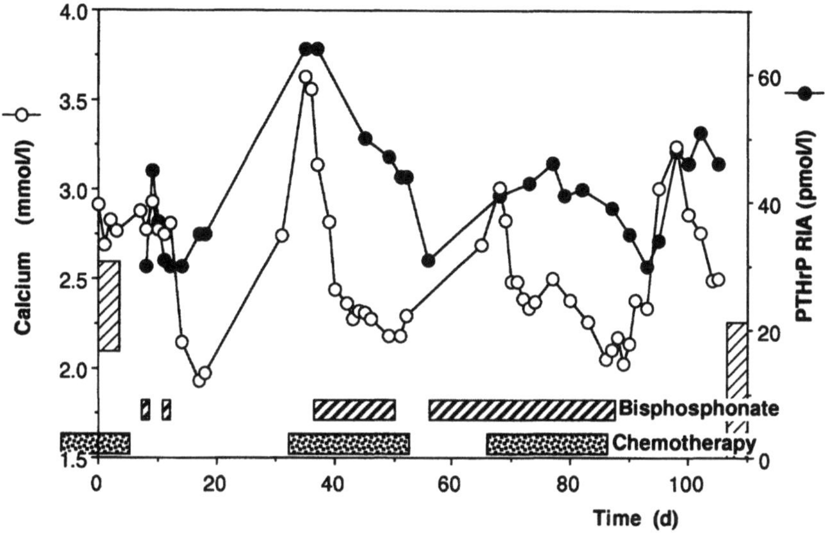

Fig. 8. Response of PTHrP levels to chemotherapy in HHM: clinical course of a 63-year-old patient with a pleuramesothelioma and hypercalcemia of malignancy. The *filled blocks* indicate peroids of therapeutic intervention to lower serum calcium either by chemotherapy or by therapy with a bisphosphonate. The changes in total serum calcium (○) and midregional PTHrP (●) concentrations are shown. The *hatched areas* indicate the normal ranges. (From Blind et al. 1993b)

calcemia (Simpson et al. 1983). There is still some controversy about the factors that may have caused elevated results in such assays.Elevated levels of PTH measured by assays specific for midregional or C-terminal fragments can either be ascribed to reduced renal clearance of these fragments (which is common in these patients) or nonspecific effects in the assay. Occasionally, some serum factor(s) (probably immunoglobulins) interact with anti-PTH antibodies and inhibit tracer binding (Mallette and Nammour 1987). Surprisingly, cross-reactivity of anti-PTH antibodies with PTHrP rarely occurs, even with antisera against the N-terminal sequence, and is excluded for midregional or C-terminal antisera, since both peptides share no homologous sequence in these regions (Fig. 2).

There are only a few well-documented cases of ectopic PTH production in the literature: PTH mRNA was found in two small cell lung tumors (Schmelzer et al. 1985; Yoshimoto et al. 1989), in an ovarial tumor (Nussbaum et al. 1990), and in a metastatic malignancy of neuroectodermal origin (Strewler et al. 1993). In two cases, PTHrP mRNA was not detectable, and PTH in plasma was increased severalfold (Nussbaum et al. 1990; Yoshimoto et al. 1989), whereas in the malignancy of neuroectodermal origin mRNA of both PTH and PTHrP was demonstrated by Northern blot, together with moderately elevated levels of PTH and PTHrP in plasma (Strewler et al. 1993). A fifth case came to our attention with proven ectopic

PTH production. This patient suffered from a bronchial carcinoid and had extremely high levels of intact PTH in plasma (253 pmol/l; normal: <6 pmol/l) (Blind et al. 1988) but normal levels of PTHrP (unpublished results). Plasma PTH and calcium fell after removal of metastatic tumor tissue, and revision of the parathyroid glands gave no pathologic result.

In lymphoproliferative malignancies, hypercalcemia is much less common than in solid neoplasms or plasmocytoma, but if present it is often associated with high levels of 1,25-dihydroxyvitamin D_3 (Adams 1989). In analogy to sarcoidosis, some lymphomas are apparently able to convert 25-hydroxyvitamin D_3 to 1,25-dihydroxyvitamin D_3, thus leading to hypercalcemia (more about the differential diagnosis can be found in the chapter by H. Schmidt-Gayk).

Several cytokines have been suspected to be involved in the syndrome of HHM. Evidence for that comes mainly from the fact that some cytokines like tumor necrosis factor α are secreted by tumors and are able to mediate bone resorption in vitro (Mundy 1990). These factors may therefore well modulate hypercalcemia in HHM (see chapter by J. Pfeilschifter), for which comes some evidence from animal studies. However, there is little evidence yet that any of these factors by itself is able to cause HHM.

Physiologic Role of PTHrP

Parathyroid hormone-related protein has now been clearly established as a major systemic factor in HHM. There is also rapidly accumulating evidence for a paracrine function of PTHrP in various tissues both in fetal life and in adults, where it is produced locally, but usually does not reach the circulation in detectable quantities. Thus, PTHrP does not seem to act as a systemic hormone in the physiology of normal adults. The one exception may be during lactation: PTHrP reaches extremely high concentrations (several orders of magnitude higher than in plasma) in breast milk (Budayr et al. 1989a), and is produced in breast tissue (Thiede and Rodan 1988) and induced by prolactin (Thiede 1989). During lactation, PTHrP is found in the circulation, and in one study it was detectable in 12 out of 19 nursing mothers (Grill et al. 1992). It has been suggested that PTHrP actually has systemic effects in this setting and thus acts as a systemic endocrine hormone (Ratcliffe 1992). Whether bioactive PTHrP from breast milk is absorbed by the newborn and may have a biological function is still controversial.

In fetal life, PTHrP seems to have a systemic function: There is evidence that PTHrP secreted by the fetal parathyroid glands maintains relative fetal hypercalcemia by stimulating transplacental calcium transport (Abbas et al. 1990; Rodda et al. 1988).

Parathyroid hormone-related protein is locally produced in several different tissues, where it may have different physiological functions. The huge number of recent papers about this question makes it impossible to give here an exhaustive summary of the role of PTHrP in normal tissue function, which is the topic of a recent review (Strewler and Nissenson 1994). Among other tissues, PTHrP seems to be involved in skin differentiation (Hayman et al. 1989; Wysolmerski et al. 1993), vascular smooth muscle regulation (Nickols et al. 1989; Winquist et al. 1987), regulation of the myometrium smooth muscle during pregnancy (Thiede et al. 1990, 1991), and chondrogenesis and mineralization of cartilage. The latter function was clearly established recently by knocking out the PTHrP gene in mice: Animals homocygous for the null mutation of the PTHrP gene did not express PTHrP and had a 100% perinatal mortality, accompanied only by obvious defects in the skeletal system, such as defective enchondral bone formation and premature mineralization (Karaplis et al. 1992).

One study found that stimulation of transplacental calcium transport by PTHrP was stimulated by the midregional (75–84) sequence and not by the N-terminal fragment of the protein as most other known effects (Care et al. 1990). This was, however, not the case in another system (Barlet et al. 1990). Furthermore, a C-terminal fragment of PTHrP (107–111) reportedly was a potent inhibitor of osteoclastic bone resorption (Fenton et al. 1991), although this finding has been controversial (Sone et al. 1992). If correct, the exciting implication of the presence of specific effects of PTHrP fragments not containing the N-terminus obviously is the existence of unique PTHrP receptors in these cells. Thus, PTHrP, discovered by its hypercalcemic effect in cancer, might lead the way to the recognition of an unexpected family of regulatory peptides.

References

Abbas SK, Pickard DW, Illingworth D, Storer J. Purdie DW, Moniz C, Dixit M, Caple IW, Ebeling PR, Rodda CP et al. (1990) Measurement of parathyroid hormone-related protein in extracts of fetal parathyroid glands and placental membranes. J Endocrinol 124:319–325

Abou-Samra AB, Jüppner H, Force T, Freeman MW, Kong XF, Schipani E, Urena P, Richards J, Bonventre JV, Potts JT Jr, Kronenberg HM, Segre GV (1992) Expression cloning of a common receptor for parathyroid hormone and parathyroid hormone-related peptide from rat osteoblast-like cells: a single receptor stimulates intracellular accumulation of both cAMP and inositol trisphosphates and increases intracellular free calcium. Proc Natl Acad Sci USA 89:2732–2736

Adams J (1989) Vitamin D metabolite-mediated hypercalcemia. Endocrinol Metabol Clin North Am 18:765–778

Barlet JP, Davicco MJ, Coxam V (1990) Synthetic parathyroid hormone-related peptide (1–34) fragment stimulates placental calcium transfer in ewes. J Endocrinol 127:33–37

Bilezikian JP (1990) Parathyroid hormone-related peptide in sickness and in health (editorial). N Engl J Med 322:1151–1153

Bilezikian JP (1991) Measurement of parathyroid hormone-related peptide in the circulation. Trends Endocrinol Metab 2:1–3

Blind E, Schmidt-Gayk H, Scharla S, Flentje D, Fischer S, Göhring U, Hitzler W (1988) Two-site assay of intact parathyroid hormone in the investigation of primary hyperparathyroidism and other disorders of calcium metabolism compared with a midregion assay. J Clin Endocrinol Metab 67:353–360

Blind E, Raue F, Götzmann J, Schmidt-Gayk H, Kohl B, Ziegler R (1992) Circulating levels of midregional parathyroid hormone-related protein in hypercalcaemia of malignancy. Clin Endocrinol (Oxf) 37:290–297

Blind E, Raue F, Knappe V, Schroth J, Ziegler R (1993a) Cyclic AMP formation in rat bone and kidney cells is stimulated equally by parathyroid hormone-related protein (PTHrP) 1–34 and PTH 1–34. Exp Clin Endocrinol 101:150–155

Blind E, Raue F, Meinel T, Bucher M, Manegold C, Ebert W, Vogt-Moykopf I, Ziegler R (1993b) Levels of parathyroid hormone-related protein in hypercalcemia of malignancy: comparison of midregional radioimmunoassay and two-site immunoradiometric assay. Clin Invest 71:31–36

Blind E, Raue F, Meinel T, Pecherstorfer M, Räth U, Schmidt-Gayk H, Kohl B, Ziegler R (1993c) Diagnostische Bedeutung von Parathormone-related-Protein bei Tumorpatienten mit Hypercalcämie. Dtsch Med Wochenschr 118:330–335

Blind E, Raue F, Meinel T, Wüster C, Ziegler R (1993d) Levels of parathyroid hormone-related protein (PTHrP) in hypercalcemia of malignancy are not lowered by treatment with the bisphosphonate BM 21.0955. Horm Metab Res 25:40–44

Budayr AA, Halloran BP, King JC, Diep D, Nissenson RA, Strewler GJ (1989a) High levels of a parathyroid hormone-like protein in milk. Proc Natl Acad Sci USA 86:7183–7185

Budayr AA, Nissenson RA, Klein RF, Pun KK, Clark OH, Diep D, Arnaud CD, Strewler GJ (1989b) Increased serum levels of a parathyroid hormone-like protein in malignancy-associated hypercalcemia. Ann Intern Med 111:807–812

Bundred NJ, Ratcliffe WA, Walker RA, Coley S, Morrison JM, Ratcliffe JG (1991) Parathyroid hormone related protein and hypercalcemia in breast cancer. Br Med J 303:1506–1509

Burtis WJ (1992) Parathyroid hormone-related protein: structure, function, and measurement. Clin Chem 38:2171–2183

Burtis WJ, Wu T, Bunch C, Wysolmerski JJ, Insogna KL, Weir EC, Broadus AE, Stewart AF (1987) Identification of a novel 17000-dalton parathyroid hormone-like adenylate cyclase-stimulating protein from a tumor associated with humoral hypercalcemia of malignancy. J Biol Chem 262:7151–7156

Burtis WJ, Brady TG, Orloff JJ, Ersbak JB, Warrell RJ, Olson Br, Wu TL, Mitnick ME, Broadus AE, Stewart AF (1990) Immunochemical characterization of circulating parathyroid hormone-related protein in patients with humoral hypercalcemia of cancer. N Engl J Med 322:1106–1112

Burtis WJ, Fodero J, Gaich G, Debeyssey M, Stewart A (1992) Preliminary characterization of circulating amino- and carboxy-terminal fragments of parathyroid hormone-related peptide in humoral hypercalcemia of malignancy. J Clin Endocrinol Metab 75:1110–1114

Care AD, Abbas SK, Pickard DW, Barri M, Drinkhill M, Findlay JB, White IR, Caple IW (1990) Stimulation of ovine placental transport of calcium and magnesium by mid-molecule fragments of human parathyroid hormone-related protein. Exp Physiol 75:605–608

Civitelli R, Martin TJ, Fausto A, Gunsten SL, Hruska KA, Avioli LV (1989) Parathyroid hormone-related peptide transiently increases cytosolic calcium in osteoblast-like cells: comparison with parathyroid hormone. Endocrinology 125:1204–1210

de Papp A, Yang K, Soifer N, Bellantoni M, Insogna K, Burtis W, Philbrick W, Stewart AF (1993) Identification of a novel C-terminal secretory form of par-

athyroid hormone-related protein. 75th annual meeting, the Endocrine society, Las Vegas, pp 545 (abstract 1978)
Deftos LJ, Hogue AR, Chalberg C, Tu S (1989) PTHrP secretion is stimulated by CT and inhibited by CgA peptides. Endocrinology 125:563–565
Dodwell DJ, Abbas SK, Morton AR, Howell A (1991) Parathyroid hormone-related protein(50–69) and response to pamidronate therapy for tumour-induced hypercalcemia. Eur J Cancer 27:1629–1633
Fenton A, Kemp B, Kent G, Moseley J, Zheng M, Rowe D, Britto J, Martin T, Nicholson G (1991) A carboxyl-terminal peptide from the parathyroid hormone-related protein inhibits bone resorption by osteoclasts. Endocrinology 129:1762–1768
Fraher LJ, Hodsman AB, Jonas K, Saunders D, Rose CI, Henderson JE, Hendy GN, Goltzman D (1992) A comparison of the in vivo biochemical responses to exogenous parathyroid hormone-(1–34) [PTH-(1–34)] and PTH-related peptide-(1–34) in man. J Clin Endocrinol Metab 75:417–423
Fukumoto S, Matsumoto T, Ikeda K, Yamashita T, Watanabe T, Yamaguchi K, Kiyokawa T, Takatsuki K, Shibuya N, Ogata E (1988) Clinical evaluation of calcium metabolism in adult T-cell leukemia/lymphoma. Arch Intern Med 148:921–925
Fukumoto S, Matsumoto T, Yamoto H, Kawashima H, Ueyama Y, Tamaoki N, Ogata E (1989) Suppression of serum 1,25-dihydroxyvitamin D is caused by elaboration of a factor that inhibits renal 1,25-dihydroxyvitamin D_3 production. Endocrinology 124:2057–2062
Grill V, Ho P, Body JJ, Johanson N, Lee SC, Kukreja SC, Moseley J, Martin TJ (1991) Parathyroid hormone related protein: elevated levels in both humoral hypercalcemia of malignancy and hypercalcemia complicating metastatic breast cancer. J Clin Endocrinol Metab 73:1309–1315
Grill V, Hillary J, Ho PM, Law FM, MacIsaac RJ, MacIsaac IA, Moseley JM, Martin TJ (1992) Parathyroid hormone-related protein: a possible endocrine function in lactation. Clin Endocrinol (Oxf) 37:405–410
Gurney H, Kefford R, Stuart-Harris R (1989) Renal phosphate threshold and response to pamidronate in humoral hypercalcemia of malignancy. Lancet ii:241–244
Hayman JA, Danks JA, Ebeling PR, Moseley JM, Kemp BE, Martin TJ (1989) Expression of parathyroid hormone related protein in normal skin and in tumours of skin and skin appendages. J Pathol 158:293–296
Heath DA (1993) Parathyroid hormone related protein. Clin Endocrinol (Oxf) 38:135–136
Henderson JE, Shustik C, Kremer R, Rabbani SA, Hendy GN, Goltzman D (1990) Circulating concentrations of parathyroid hormone-like peptide in malignancy and in hyperparathyroidism. J Bone Miner Res 5:105–113
Horiuchu N, Caulfield MP, Fisher JE, Goldman ME, McKee RL, Reagen JE, Levy JJ, Nutt RF, Schofield TL, Clemens TL, Rosenblatt M (1987) Similarity of synthetic peptide from human tumor to PTH in vivo and in vitro. Science 238: 1566–1568
Ikeda K, Lu C, Weir EC, Mangin M Broadus AE (1989) Transcriptional regulation of the parathyroid hormone-related peptide gene by glucocorticoids and vitamin D in a human C-cell line. J Biol Chem 264:15743–15746
Jüppner H, Abou-Samra A, Uneno S, Gu WX, Potts JT Jr, Segre GV (1988) The parathyroid hormone-like peptide associated with humoral hypercalcemia of malignancy and parathyroid hormone bind to the same receptor on the plasma membrane of ROS 17/2.8 cells. J Biol Chem 263:8557–8560
Kao PC, Klee GG, Taylor RL, Heath H III (1990) Parathyroid hormone-related peptide in plasma of patients with hypercalcemia and malignant lesions. Mayo Clin Proc 65:1399–1407

Karaplis A, Tybulewicz V, Mulligan R, Kronenberg H (1992) Disruption of parathyroid hormone-related peptide gene leads to a multitude of skeletal abnormalities and perinatal mortality. J Bone Miner Res 7[Suppl 1]:S93 (abstract 1)
Kemp BE, Moseley JM, Rodda CP, Ebeling PR, Wettenhall REH, Stapleton D, Diefenbach JH, Ure F, Michelangeli VP, Simmons HA, Raisz LG, Martin TJ (1987) Parathyroid hormone-related protein of malignancy: active synthetic fragments. Science 238:1568–1570
Mallette L, Nammour H (1987) False-positive elevations of midregional parathyroid hormone: inhibition of radioligand binding by a heterophilic antibody in patient serum. In: Cohn D, Martin T, Meunier P (eds) Calcium regulation and bone metabolism, basic and clinical aspects. Excerpta Medica, Amsterdam, pp 550
Mangin M, Ikeda K, Dreyer BE, Milstone L, Broadus AE (1988a) Two distinct tumor-derived, parathyroid hormone-like peptides result from alternative ribonucleic acid splicing. Mol Endocrinol 2:1049–1055
Mangin M, Webb AC, Dreyer BE, Posillico JT, Ikeda K, Weir EC, Stewart AF, Bander NH, Milstone L, Barton DE, Franke U, Broadus AE (1988b) Identification of a cDNA encoding a parathyroid hormone-like peptide from a human tumor associated with humoral hypercalcemia of malignancy. Proc Natl Acad Sci USA 85:597–601
Mangin M, Ikeda K, Dreyer BE, Broadus AE (1989) Isolation and characterization of the human parathyroid hormone-like peptide gene. Proc Natl Acad Sci USA 86:2408–2412
Mangin M, Ikeda K, Broadus AE (1990) Structure of the mouse gene encoding parathyroid hormone-related peptide. Gene 95:195–202
Mitlak BH, Hutchinson JS, Kaufman SD, Nussbaum SR (1991) Parathyroid hormone-related peptide mediates hypercalcemia in an islet cell tumor of the pancreas. Horm Metab Res 23:344–346
Moseley JM, Kubota M, Diefenbach JH, Wettenhall RE, Kemp BE, Suva LJ, Rodda CP, Ebeling PR, Hudson PJ, Zajac JD, Martin TJ (1987) Parathyroid hormone-related protein purified from a human lung cancer cell line. Proc Natl Acad Sci USA 84:5048–5052
Motokura T, Fukumoto S, Takahashi S, Watanabe T, Matsumoto T, Igarashi T, Ogata E (1988) Expression of parathyroid hormone – related protein in a human T cell lymphotrophic virus type I-infected T cell line. Biochem Biophys Res Commun 154:1182–1188
Mundy GR (1985) Pathogenesis of hypercalcemia of malignancy. Clin Endocrinol 23:705–714
Mundy G (1990) Malignancy and hypercalcemia – humoral hypercalcemia of malignancy, hypercalcemia associated with osteolytic metastasis. In: Mundy G (ed) Calcium homeostasis: hypercalcemia and hypocalcemia. Dunitz, London, pp 69–99
Nickols GA, Nana AD, Nickols MA, DiPette DJ, Asimakis GK (1989) Hypotension and cardiac stimulation due to the parathyroid hormone-related protein, humoral hypercalcemia of malignancy factor. Endocrinology 125:834–841
Nissenson RA, Diep D, Strewler GJ (1988) Synthetic peptides comprising the amino-terminal sequence of a parathyroid hormone-like protein from human malignancies. Binding to parathyroid hormone receptors and activation of adenylate cyclase in bone cells and kidney. J Biol Chem 263:12866–12871
Nussbaum SR, Gaz RD, Arnold A (1990) Hypercalcemia and ectopic secretion of parathyroid hormone by an ovarian carcinoma with rearrangement of the gene for parathyroid hormone. N Engl J Med 323:1324–1328
Orloff JJ, Wu TL, Heath HW, Brady TG, Brines ML, Stewart AF (1989) Characterization of canine renal receptors for the parathyroid hormone-like protein associated with humoral hypercalcemia of malignancy. J Biol Chem 264:6097–6103

Pandian MR, Morgan CH, Carlton E, Segre GV (1992) Modified immunoradiometric assay of parathyroid hormone-related protein: clinical application in the differential diagnosis of hypercalcemia. Clin Chem 38:282–288

Powell GJ, Southby J, Danks JA, Stillwell RG, Hayman JA, Henderson MA, Bennett RC, Martin TJ (1991) Localization of parathyroid hormone-related protein in breast cancer metastases: increased incidence in bone compared with other sites. Cancer Res 51:3059–3061

Ralston SH, Gardner MD, Dryburgh FJ, Cowan RA, Jenkins AS, Boyle IT (1985) Comparison of aminohydroxypropylidene diphosphonate, mithramycin and corticosteroids/calcitonin in treatment of cancer associated hypercalcaemia. Lancet ii:907–910

Ralston SH, Gardner MD, Jenkins AS, McKillop JH, Boyle IT (1987) Malignancy-associated hypercalcaemia: relationship between mechanisms of hypercalcaemia and response to antihypercalcemic therapy. Bone Miner 2:227–242

Ratcliffe WA (1992) Role of parathyroid hormone-related protein in lactation. Clin Endocrinol (Oxf) 37:402–404

Ratcliffe WA, Ratcliffe JG (1990) Parathyroid hormone-related protein. In: Schmidt-Gayk H, Armbruster FP, Bouillon R (eds) Calcium regulating hormones, vitamin D metabolites, and cyclic AMP assays and their clinical application. Springer, Berlin Heidelberg New York, pp 213–227

Ratcliffe WA, Norbury S, Heath DA, Ratcliffe JG (1991a) Development and validation of an immunoradiometric assay of parathyrin-related protein in unextracted plasma. Clin Chem 37:678–685

Ratcliffe WA, Norbury S, Stott RA, Heath DA, Ratcliffe JG (1991b) Immunoreactivity of plasma parathyrin-related peptide: three region-specific radioimmunoassays and a two-site immunoradiometric assay compared. Clin Chem 37:1781–1787

Rizzoli R, Bonjour JP (1989) High extracellular calcium increases the production of a parathyroid hormone-like activity by cultured Leydig tumor cells associated with humoral hypercalcemia. J Bone Miner Res 4:839–844

Rizzoli R, Caverzasio J, Chapuy MC, Martin TJ, Bonjour JP (1989) Role of bone and kidney in parathyroid hormone-related peptide-induced hypercalcemia in rats. J Bone Miner Res 4:759–765

Rodan SB, Noda M, Wesolowski G, Rosenblatt M, Rodan GA (1988) Comparison of postreceptor effects of 1–34 human hypercalcemia factor and 1–34 human parathyroid hormone in rat osteosarcoma cells. J Clin Invest 81:927–927

Rodda CP, Kubota M, Heath JA, Ebeling PR, Moseley JM, Care AD, Caple IW, Martin TJ (1988) Evidence for a novel parathyroid hormone-related protein in fetal lamb parathyroid glands and sheep placenta: comparisons with a similar protein implicated in humoral hypercalcaemia of malignancy. J Endocrinol 117:261–271

Scharla SH, Pecherstorfer M, Lempert UG, Minne HW, Sarrach M, Baumgartner G, Ziegler R (1991) PTH-related protein (PTHrP) im Serum von Patienten mit Tumorhyperkalzämie. Med Klin 86:186–189

Schilling T, Pecherstorfer M, Blind E, Leidig G, Ziegler R, Raue F (1993) Parathyroid hormone-related protein (PTHrP) does not regulate 1,25-dihydroxyvitamin D serum levels in hypercalcemia of malignancy. J Clin Endocrinol Metab 76: 801–803

Schipani E, Karga H, Karaplis A, Potts JT Jr, Kronenberg H, Segre GV, Abou-Samra A, Jüppner H (1993) Identical complementary deoxyribonucleic acids encode a human renal and bone parathyroid hormone (PTH)/PTH-related peptide receptor. Endocrinology 132:2157–2165

Schmelzer H, Hesch R, Mayer H (1985) Parathyroid hormone and PTH mRNA in a human small cell lung cancer. In: Havemann K, Sorenson G, Gropp C (eds)

Peptide hormones in lung cancer. Springer, Berlin Heidelberg New York, pp 88–93

Simpson EL, Mundy GR, D'Souza SM, Ibbotson KJ, Bockman R, Jacobs JW (1983) Absence of parathyroid hormone messenge RNA in nonparathyroid tumors associated with hypercalcemia. N Engl J Med 309:325–330

Soifer NE, Stewart AF (1992) Measurement of PTH-related protein and the role of PTH-related protein in malignancy-asociated hypercalcemia. In: Halloran BP, Nissenson RA (eds) Parathyroid hormone-related protein: normal physiology and its role in cancer. CRC Press, Boca Raton, pp 93–143

Sone T, Kohno H, Kikuchi H, Ikeda T, Kasai R, Kikuchi Y, Takeuchi R, Konishi J, Shigeno C (1992) Human parathyroid hormone-related peptide-(107–111) does not inhibit bone resorption in neonatal mouse calvariae. Endocrinology 131:2742–2746

Southby J, Kissin MW, Danks JA, Hayman JA, Moseley JM, Henderson MA, Bennett RC, Martin TJ (1990) Immunohistochemical localization of parathyroid hormone-related protein in human breast cancer. Cancer Res 50:7710–7716

Stewart A, Vignery A, Silverglate A et al. (1982) Quantitative bone histomorphometry in humoral hypercalcemia of malignancy: uncoupling of bone cell activity. J Clin Endocrinol Metab 55:219–227

Stewart AF, Horst R, Deftos LJ, Cadman EC, Lang R, Broadus AE (1980) Biochemical evaluation of patients with cancer-associated hypercalcemia: evidence for humoral and non-humoral groups. N Engl J Med 303:1377–1383

Stewart AF, Mangin M, Wu T, Goumas D, Insogna KL, Burtis WJ, Broadus AE (1988) A synthetic human parathyroid hormone-like protein stimulates bone resorption and causes hypercalcemia in rats. J Clin Invest 81:596–600

Strewler G, Budayr A, Clark O, Nissenson R (1993a) Production of parathyroid hormone by a malignant nonparathyroid tumor in a hypercalcemic patient. J Clin Endocrinol Metab 76:1373–1375

Strewler GJ, Nissenson RA (1994) The parathyroid hormone-related protein as a regulator of normal tissue functions. In: Kohler PO (ed) Current opinion in endocrinology and diabetes. Current Science, Philadelphia, pp 286–292

Strewler GJ, Stern PH, Jacobs JW, Eveloff J, Klein RF, Leung SC, Rosenblatt M, Nissenson RA (1987) Parathyroid hormone-like protein from human renal carcinoma cells. Structural and functional homology with parathyroid hormone. J Clin Invest 80:1803–1807

Suva LJ, Winslow GA, Wettenhall RE, Hammonds RG, Moseley JM, Diefenbach-Jagger H, Rodda CP, Kemp BE, Rodriguez H, Chen EY, Hudson PJ, Martin TJ, Wood WI (1987) A parathyroid hormone-related protein implicated in malignant hypercalcemia: cloning and expression. Science 237:893–896

Suva LJ, Mather KA, Gillespie MT, Webb GC, Ng KW, Winslow GA, Wood WI, Martin TJ, Hudson PJ (1989) Structure of the 5′ flanking region of the gene encoding human parathyroid-hormone-related protein (PTHrP). Gene 77:95–105

Thiede MA (1989) The mRNA encoding a parathyroid hormone-like peptide is produced in mammary tissue in response to elevations in serum prolactin. Mol Endocrinol 3:1443–1447

Thiede MA, Rodan GA (1988) Expression of a calcium-mobilizing parathyroid hormone-like peptide in lactating mammary tissue. Science 242:278–280

Thiede MA, Strewler GJ, Nissenson RA, Rosenblatt M, Rodan GA (1988) Human renal carcinoma expresses two messages encoding a parathyroid hormone-like peptide: evidence for the alternative splicing of a single-copy gene. Proc Natl Acad Sci USA 85:4605–4609

Thiede MA, Daifotis AG, Weir EC, Brines ML, Burtis WJ, Ikeda K, Dreyer BE, Garfield RE, Broadus AE (1990) Intrauterine occupancy controls expression of the parathyroid hormone-related peptide gene in preterm rat myometrium. Proc Natl Acad Sci USA 87:6969–6973

Thiede MA, Harm SC, Hasson DM, Gardner RM (1991) In vivo regulation of parathyroid hormone-related peptide messenger ribonucleic acid in the rat uterus by 17 beta-estradiol. Endocrinology 128:2317–2323

Wagner H, Blind E, Raue F (1993) Secretion and storage of parathyroid hormone-related protein is decreased by vitamin D and glucocorticoids in a C-cell line and in the rat Walker carcinosarcoma 256. Exp Clin Endocrinol 101[Suppl 1]:174 (abstract 300)

Winquist RJ, Baskin EP, Vlasuk GP (1987) Synthetic tumor-derived human hypercalcemic factor exhibits parathyroid hormone-like vasorelaxation in renal arteries. Biochem Biophys Res Commun 149:227–232

Wu TL, Soifer NE, Burtis WJ, Milstone LM, Stewart AF (1991) Glycosylation of parathyroid hormone-related peptide secreted by human epidermal keratinocytes. J Clin Endocrinol Metab 73:1002–1007

Wysolmerski J, Philbrick W, Zhou J, Broadus A, Milstone L (1993) Overexpression of parathyroid hormone-related peptide in skin causes abnormal hair growth, hyperkeratosis, and abnormal pigmentation. 75th Annual Meeting, The Endocrine Society, Las Vegas, p 544 (abstract 1976)

Yamada H, Tsutsumi M, Fukase M, Fujimori A, Yamamoto Y, Miyauchi A, Fujii Y, Noda T, Fujii N, Fujita T (1989) Effects of human PTH-related peptide and human PTH on cyclic AMP production and cytosolic free calcium in an osteoblastic cell clone. Bone Miner 6:45–54

Yasuda T, Banville D, Hendy GN, Goltzman D (1989) Characterization of the human parathyroid hormone-like peptide gene. Functional and evolutionary aspects. J Biol Chem 264:7720–7725

Yoshimoto K, Yamasaki R, Sakai H, Tezuka U, Takahashi M, Iizuka M, Sekiya T, Saito S (1989) Ectopic production of parathyroid hormone by small cell lung cancer in a patient with hypercalcemia. J Clin Endocrinol Metab 68:976–981

In Vivo Models of Hypercalcemia of Malignancy

T. Schilling

Department of Internal Medicine I – Endocrinology and Metabolism, University of Heidelberg, Bergheimerstraße 58, 69115 Heidelberg, Germany

Introduction

For about 30 years there has been interest in animal models of hypercalcemia of malignancy (HHM), which affects not only humans but also animals. Dogs for example spontaneously develop hypercalcemia with malignant diseases such as lymphosarcoma (Weller and Melcon 1978; Heath et al. 1980) and adenocarcinoma (Patnaik et al. 1978). This was especially observed with adenocarcinoma derived from the apocrine gland of the anal sac (Meuten et al. 1981, 1982a,b). Hypercalcemia also occurs in cats, but more rarely than in dogs (Engelman et al. 1985; Chew and Carothers 1989; Klausner et al. 1990). There are even reports of hypercalcemia in horses bearing solid malignant tumors (McCoy and Beasley 1986).

Animal models for HHM have received increasing attention for several reasons. Because patients suffering from HHM are usually severely ill, efforts to investigate the underlying pathophysiologic mechanisms are often limited. Therefore investigators have been looking to animal models for a better understanding of the mechanisms of humoral hypercalcemia, both in vivo and in vitro. Particularly new forms of therapy have often been tested using these models. Another advantage of animal models is that the hypercalcemia develops over a relatively short period of time. Furthermore, animal-derived tumor tissues and malignant cells grown in tissue culture serve as important sources for the isolation of the responsible factor/factors of the hypercalcemia and for the examination of its pathophysiologic regulation in vitro. There are several models for the induction of HHM in animals under experimental conditions:

1. Induction of a tumor by drugs
2. Allogeneic transplantation of tumors
3. Xenogeneic transplantion of tumors into normal or immunodeficient animals
4. Infusion of the possible responsible factor/factors of HHM

Not every model may serve as a paradigm for the human HHM. Although most of the models to be described share many of the in vivo features of the human syndrome, there are distinct differences between the human and the animal syndrome which must be considered.

Animal Models: Overview

Rats, mice and rabbits are used for experimental induction of HHM. In addition, spontaneously developing HHM in dogs has often been examined in order to answer questions about the syndrome.

Table 1 gives an overview of the established rat models. Both Leydig cell tumor (Rice et al. 1971, 1975) and Walker carcinosarcoma 256 (Hilgard et al. 1970; Minne et al. 1975) are tumors derived from neoplasms which have spontaneously developed in rats. The dark agouti rat mammary adenocarcinoma is a recently characterized tumor, which can readily be maintained in tissue culture and which causes hypercalcemia, anemia and hypoglycemia when retransplanted into the host (Coyle et al. 1990).

In contrast to the allogeneic transplantation, there are models in which xenogeneic transplantion from human tumors into athymic nude rats is employed (Ikeda et al. 1988). Another possibility is the induction of mammary tumors in rats, by injection of nitrosurea compounds (Gullino et al. 1975). This model, in which the rat develops hypercalcemia in 92%, mimics human breast carcinoma more closely than any other available tumor model (Stoica et al. 1983). Since the successful isolation and synthesis of parathyroid hormone-related protein (PTHrP), one of the responsible factors for HHM, it is possible to cause hypercalcemia by infusion of synthetic PTHrP (Thompson et al. 1988).

Table 2 summarizes the currently applied mice models. In contrast to the described rat models, there are only few allogeneic and many xenogeneic

Table 1. Rat models of humoral hypercalcemia of malignancy (HHM)

Model	Abbreviation	Transplantation	Species	Tumor origin
Walker carcinosarcoma 256	WCS 256	Allogeneic	Rat	Mammary gland
Rice-500 Leydig cell tumor	Leydig	Allogeneic	Rat	Testis
Mammary adenocarcinoma	Dark agouti	Allogeneic	Rat	Mammary gland
Induced mammary carcinoma	–	Injection of nitrosourea compounds	Rat	Mammary gland
Transplantation in immunodeficient rats	–	Xenogeneic	Nude rat	Human
Infusion of PTHrP	–	–	Rat	–

Table 2. Mice models of humoral hypercalcemia of malignancy (HHM)

Model	Transplantation	From species	To species	Tumor origin
$HSDM_1$ mouse fibrosarcoma	Allogeneic	Mice	Normal mice	Fibrosarcoma
CE mammary carcinoma	Allogeneic	Mice	Normal mice	Mammary gland
Squamous cell carcinoma	Induction by dimethylbenzanthracene	Mice	Normal mice	Skin
Infusion of cytokines	Synthesized PTHrP	Human	Normal mice	–
Transplantation of transfected cells into athymic mice	Xenogeneic	Chinese hamster	Nude mice	Ovarian cells
Canine adenocarcinoma (CAC8, CAC9)	Xenogeneic	Dog	Nude mice	Anal sac
Transplantation of human tumors into athymic mice	Xenogeneic	Human	Nude mice	Rhabdomyosarcoma Renal carcinoma Prostate carcinoma Ascites sarcoma Pancreatic carcinoma Transitional cell carcinoma (TCC) Bladder carcinoma Mammary carcinoma Anaplastic lung cancer Esophageal carcinoma Squamous cell carcinoma

transplantation models in mice. Allogeneic models, which use normal mice as host animals, are the inducible transplantable $HSDM_1$ mouse fibrosarcoma (Goldhaber 1960) and the CE mammary carcinoma (Delmonte et al. 1966; Barrett et al. 1978). Two further models are the induction of cutaneous squamous cell carcinoma by painting with dimethylbenzanthracene (Gkonos et al. 1984) and the infusion of synthesized PTHrP (Yates et al. 1988; Rosol et al. 1988; Nagasaki et al. 1989). With the development of a strain of immunodeficient mice, designated nude mice, it became possible to transplant a variety of tumors from other species into these animals (Salomon et al. 1980). Tumors transplanted into nude mice to induce HHM are rhabdomyosarcoma (Takeuchi et al. 1982), renal carcinoma (Strewler et al. 1983, 1986; Klein et al. 1987; Weir et al. 1988b), prostate carcinoma (Linehan et al. 1986), ascites sarcoma (Suzuki and Yamada 1991), pancreatic carcinoma (Nagata et al. 1989), transitional-cell carcinoma (Bringhurst et al. 1986), bladder carcinoma (Nemoto et al. 1988), mammary carcinoma (Lee and Baylink 1983), anaplastic lung cancer (Anger et al. 1982; Linkhart et al. 1989), esophageal cancer (Sato et al. 1989a), and squamous cell carcinoma (Saito et al. 1981; Abramson et al. 1984; Kukreja et al. 1988a; Shipley et al. 1988), the latter being the most relevant model system.

Another tumor for xenogeneic transplantation is the canine adenocarcinoma (CAC); it was first described by Rosol and coworkers (Rosol et al. 1986a,b). A newly developed model using nude mice, applied by Mundy and his group, is the transplantation of Chinese hamster ovarian cells transfected with genes for different cytokines such as interleukin-6 (Black et al. 1991), tumor necrosis factor (Johnson et al. 1989), parathyroid hormone-related peptide (Guise et al. 1992) and transforming growth factor alpha (Yates et al. 1992). This enables each single cytokine to be tested in its pathophysiologic role in mediating the syndrome of HHM.

The VX-2 carcinoma is the only rabbit model of HHM. It originates from a papilloma (Kidd and Rous 1940), and rabbits bearing the VX-2 carcinoma develop hypercalcemia (Wilson et al. 1961, 1965).

Animal Models: In Detail

Naturally Occurring HHM in Dogs

Dogs relatively often spontaneously develop hypercalcemia of malignancy (Heath et al. 1980; Meuten et al. 1981). Adenocarcinoma of the anal sac (CAC) and lymphosarcoma are the neoplasms that most frequently cause hypercalcemia in dogs. Serum PTH levels are suppressed (Meuten et al. 1982b, 1983a,b; Heath et al. 1980; Rosol et al. 1992b) or are in the normal range (Weir et al. 1988c; Rosol et al. 1992b). All dogs show increased bone resorption (Norrdin and Powers 1983) accompanied by unchanged bone formation parameters (Weir et al. 1988c). Urinary cAMP, calcium and phosphorus excretion is increased (Weir et al. 1988c; Meuten et al. 1983b). In dogs with CAC, PTHrP plays an important role in the induction of hypercalcemia. Rosol et al. (1992b) reported a significant positive correlation between serum PTHrP and serum calcium. The role of prostaglandins is controversial. Although Meuten et al. (1983b) found elevated 15-keto-prostaglandin E_2 in dogs with lymphosarcoma, other studies did not confirm these results (Meuten et al. 1983a; Heath et al. 1980).

Whether 1,25-dihydroxyvitamin D [1,25-$(OH)_2D$] is of importance in the mediation of HHM in dogs is still unclear. Meuten et al. (1983b) found suppressed 1,25-$(OH)_2D$ levels whereas others found normal (Weir et al. 1988c; Meuten et al. 1982b, 1983a) or even elevated 1,25$(OH)_2D$ levels (Rosol et al. 1992b). There was no significant correlation between 1,25-$(OH)_2D$ and calcium or 1,25-$(OH)_2D$ and PTHrP (Rosol et al. 1992b). These findings are in contrast to human HHM, where 1,25-$(OH)_2D$ is suppressed.

Walker Carcinosarcoma 256 (WCS 256) in Rats

The 256 strain has received the most attention of several variants of the Walker carcinosarcoma (WCS). The WCS 256 arose spontaneously in the region of the mammary gland of a pregnant albino rat (Stewart et al. 1959). The WCS cells were thought to originate from epithelial cells, but Simpkins et al. (1991) showed that the rat WCS cell lines are hematopoietic in origin with the absence of cells with epithelial cell markers. There are two variants of the WCS 256, line A and B. Line A does not cause hypercalcemia whereas line B leads to the syndrome of HHM (D'Souza et al. 1984c; Guaitani et al. 1985).

The tumor consistently produces hypercalcemia over a period of 5–9 days. After tumor removal the serum calcium level normalizes. Hypercalcemia has been shown to occur despite parathyroidectomy in tumor-bearing animals (Hilgard et al. 1970; Minne et al. 1975). The WCS causes osteoclasia and increased bone resorption, both in vivo (Schäfer et al. 1976; Schmidt-Gayk et al. 1979) and in vitro (Rodan et al. 1983). The tumor-bearing animals develop hypophosphatemia and calcinosis. In addition to the increased bone resorption, altered renal calcium handling seems to play a key role in the hypercalcemia associated with this HHM model (Schmidt-Gayk et al. 1979; Hurtado et al. 1988, 1991). Accompanying anorexia is characteristic for the syndrome of HHM. Steele and coworkers (1988) found that marginal deficits of hypothalamic dynorphin, which coincide with the phase of tumor-induced anorexia, might contribute to the reduction in food intake.

There is great evidence that parathyroid hormone-related protein (PTHrP) is the humoral factor causing hypercalcemia in the WCS 256 (Scharla et al. 1991; Torres et al. 1992; de Miguel and Esbrit 1992). We have recently shown that i.p. administration of native polyclonal antiserum against PTHrP (53–84) in rats bearing the WCS 256 leads to a significant decrease of plasma calcium. This indicates that PTHrP is not only produced by the WCS tumor but also is the causative factor in mediating hypercalcemia (Raue et al. 1993). Another cytokine playing a role in the WCS 256 syndrome is transforming growth factor-β (TGF-β) (D'Souza et al. 1984b). Orr et al. (1990) showed that TGF-β, released from resorbing bone, can influence the migratory behavior of the osteotropic WCS 256 cell line in the sense of being a chemoattractant for WCS cells to metastasize to bone.

Rice-500 Leydig Cell Tumor in Rats

This model was developed by Rice and coworkers in the 1970s. Several strains of the Leydig cell tumor exist, the H500 line being the most important. The Rice H500 tumor is a transplantable nonmetastasizing testicular tumor of Fischer rats associated with hypercalcemia, hypophosphatemia, hypercalciuria, hyperphosphaturia and increased urine cyclic adenosine monophosphate (cAMP) excretion (Troyer et al. 1982; Berger et al. 1982; Spiegel et al. 1983; Insogna et al. 1984; Saxe et al. 1985). The hypercalcemia develops within 8–10 days. The Leydig tumor-induced hypercalcemia is associated with hypertension. Although the vascular reactivity to norepinephrine is decreased, the hypertension could be due to the elevation of the vasoactive hormones norepinephrine and angiotensin (Sowers and Barrett 1982; Nyby et al. 1987). These findings are in contrast to clinical studies, in which accompanying hypotension is reported in patients suffering from HHM (Mundy 1987).

Bone metabolism in Leydig rats is characterized by osteoclasia and increased bone resorption accompanied by decreased bone formation (Tam et al. 1984). Immunoreactive parathyroid hormone (PTH) levels are found to be suppressed and 1,25-$(OH)_2D$ levels are increased (Berger et al. 1982; Insogna et al. 1984). The latter observation is likely to represent a difference in species response. In accordance with the Walker carcinosarcoma, Rizzoli and coworkers (1986) demonstrated that the Leydig cell tumor increases tubular reabsorption of calcium. This may, apart from the increased bone resorption, play an essential role in the pathogenesis of Leydig cell tumor-induced hypercalcemia. Furthermore, Sartori et al. (1988) were able to show that the renal phosphate uptake is specifically and persistently impaired, which contributes to the derangement of phosphate metabolism.

Calcitonin values and plasma prostaglandin (PGE) levels have been reported to increase during the development of hypercalcemia in rats (Berger et al. 1982). But the PGE elevation does not seem to play a significant role, as administration of indomethacin (20 mg/kg per day) did not prevent the development of hypercalcemia.

Meanwhile it has clearly been demonstrated that PTHrP is a responsible factor mediating hypercalcemia in the Leydig cell tumor. Weir et al. isolated a PTH-like protein (1988a) from the Leydig tumor, Gaich and Burtis (1990) measured circulating PTHrP in rats bearing the Leydig tumor, and Henderson and coworkers (1990) were able to normalize plasma calcium for several days by passive i.v. immunization with antiserum against PTHrP.

Other groups have amassed evidence to suggest that tumor-derived transforming growth factor is also a responsible mediator (Ibbotson et al. 1983). Ibbotson et al. showed that tumor extracts contain a single peak of bone-resorbing activity on gel filtration, which co-elutes with a peak of soft-agar colony-stimulating activity and a peak of activity demonstrating competitive displacement of EGF from its receptor (Ibbotson et al. 1985a). These two latter properties are associated with transforming growth factors. Insogna and coworkers (1987) confirmed these results by copurification of TGFβ-like with PTH-like bone-resorbing activities from the Leydig H500 tumor. The possible role of TGFβ is underlined by the fact that EGF receptor antisera block the bone-resorbing activity in tumor-conditioned medium (D'Souza et al. 1984a).

Rats bearing the Leydig cell tumor also show increased circulating immunoreactive tumor necrosis factor (TNF) (Sabatini et al. 1990). However, not the tumor cells but rather the host cells seem to produce TNF. Cultured Leydig cells stimulate TNF production by splenic mononuclear cells, by peritoneal macrophages and by peripheral blood monocytes. This TNF production may be mainly responsible for the cachexia in Leydig tumor bearing rats (Mundy 1991).

VX-2 Carcinoma of Rabbits

The VX-2 carcinoma is the result of a malignant transformation of the viral-induced Shope papilloma (Kidd and Rous 1940). Following its implantation in muscle, the carcinoma grows rapidly with local infiltration and metastases to regional lymph nodes and lungs (Voelkel et al. 1975; Young et al. 1976, 1978). Development of hypercalcemia takes a longer time interval, usually 2–4 weeks after tumor transplantation, than in the Walker carcinosarcoma and Leydig tumor model. Varying degrees of increased osteoclastic activity and increased bone resorption are evident at different skeletal sites accompanied by diminution in parameters of osteoblastic function (Hough et al. 1977; Wolfe et al. 1978). In addition to hypercalcemia, the VX-2 carcinoma also produces hypophosphatemia. In contrast to the Walker carcinosarcoma and the Leydig cell tumor in rats, serum PTH and urinary cAMP excretion do not change (Schmidt-Gayk et al. 1983).

Extracts of tumor tissue and conditioned medium from VX-2 cells grown in culture contain large amounts of prostaglandin E2 (Voelkel et al. 1975). Prostaglandins appear in the circulation before hypercalcemia and indomethacin treatment had been shown to prevent the PGE rise as well as the appearance of hypercalcemia (Voelkel et al. 1975; Tashjian et al. 1977a; Seyberth et al. 1977; Alam et al. 1980). Based on these results, it was felt that prostaglandins mediate the hypercalcemia in the VX-2 carcinoma-bearing rabbits, yet other evidence has called this conclusion into serious question. Doppelt and coworkers (1982) have shown that animals maintained on a standard dietary calcium intake became hypercalcemic and that treatment with indomethacin did not influence the level of hypercalcemia although it normalized urine excretion of prostaglandin E_2. Dietary calcium restriction promptly restored the plasma calcium to normal and treatment with oral indomethacin, beginning at day 0 of transplantation, did not prevent hypercalcemia. Bisphosphonates did not prevent the appearence of hypercalcemia in animals fed a diet high in calcium, but prevented hypercalcemia in animals fed on a calcium-free diet. These data argue that the principal mechanism of hypercalcemia in the VX-2 carcinoma is intestinal hyperabsorption of calcium rather than bone resorption and that prostaglandins may not be the main responsible factor for HHM. Which factor/factors are responsible in this model remains unclear to date.

$HSDM_1$ Fibrosarcoma in Mice

Swiss albino mice transplanted with the mouse fibrosarcoma ($HSDM_1$) develop hypercalcemia over a period of 2–3 weeks (Tashjian et al. 1977b). Additional parameters of calcium metabolism have not been examined in this model so far. Hydrocortisone and indomethacin therapy prevent hypercalcemia in tumor-bearing animals whereas a diet low in calcium has no effect on the hypercalcemia (Tashjian et al. 1973, 1977b, 1984). A significant rise in plasma levels of prostaglandin E_2 metabolites occurs before the appearance of hypercalcemia. In vitro, $HSDM_1$ cells in culture have been shown to possess bone-resorbing activity and to produce large amounts of prostaglandin E_2 (Tashjian et al. 1972, 1974; Levine et al. 1972). Coculture with indomethacin blocks both bone resorption and prostaglandin E_2 production (Levine et al. 1972). These data demonstrate convincing evidence that the elevated circulating level of prostaglandin E_2 is responsible for the mediation of the hypercalcemia. This is a seemingly rare occurrence in man. Whether other factors, like PTHrP, are responsible in this model remains open to date.

Murime Mammary Carcinoma (CE maca) in Normal Mice

When transplanted subcutaneously or intramuscularly, the CE mammary carcinoma causes hypercalcemia over 3–4 weeks, and tumor removal reverses the hypercalcemia (Barrett et al. 1978). Hypercalcemia is associated with a significant increase in urinary hydroxyproline, an increase in marrow medullary area and an increase in the number of endosteal osteoclasts, together indicating that the cause of hypercalcemia is an increase in bone resorption (Lee and Baylink 1983; Riddle et al. 1987). In parallel to the hypercalcemia, hypercalciuria and an increase in urinary cyclic AMP excretion occur.

Media from cells grown in tissue culture have been shown to induce bone resorption that can be blocked with indomethacin, suggesting that prostaglandins might play a role in mediating bone resorption (Lau and Lee 1983). However, the nature of the systemic mediator still remains unclear.

Mice bearing the CE mammary tumor develop granulocytosis. This symptom has recently been addressed in studies. There is evidence that CE mammary carcinoma cells produce factors affecting granulopoiesis and bone cells. This has been shown by in vivo and in vitro studies (Lee et al. 1987). Lee and coworkers (1989) demonstrated that granulocyte colony-stimulating factor (G-CSF) and macrophage colony-stimulating factor (M-CSF) are produced constitutively from the CE mammary cells, and that G-CSF is likely to be responsible for granulocytosis induced by this tumor.

Induction of Squamous Cell Carcinoma in Normal Mice

In 1984 Gkonos and coworkers reported the induction of a squamous cell carcinoma in mice by painting the skin with dimethylbenzanthracene. Ninety percent of the animals developed HHM, which, with the exception of elevated plasma 1,25-$(OH)_2D$ levels, mimics the human syndrome. The mice developed hypercalcemia, hypophosphatemia, hypercalciuria, suppressed PTH levels, elevated urinary cAMP and accelerated bone resorption (Gkonos et al. 1984). Extracts from the tumor tissue were found to contain adenylate cyclase-stimulating activity (ACSA), which was only partly inhibited by the competitive PTH antagonist (3–34)bPTH amide. Burtis and coworkers (1986) found that this adenylate cyclase-stimulating activity can be resolved into two distinct fractions. One fraction contained activity apparently interacting specifically with the PTH receptor, suggesting that this fraction contains PTHrP, while the other peak appeared to be acting independently of the PTH receptor. These two different adenylate cyclase-stimulating activities distinguish this model from the human syndrome. The responsible factor has not definitively been established to date.

Canine Adenocarcinoma (CAC) in Nude Mice

Two tumor lines, CAC-8 and CAC-9, exist; the first being the one more often used. It grows as a subcutaneous neoplasm in nude mice. As Rosol et al. (1986a) demonstrated, nude mice with transplanted CAC-8 develop hypercalcemia and moderate hypophosphatemia without bone metastases. Urinary excretion of calcium, cAMP and hydroxyproline and the rate of bone resorption as well as bone formation were increased. In contrast to other animal models of HHM, the CAC-8 model shows a slow progressive growth rate and a slow development of hypercalcemia about 4–5 weeks after transplantation (Rosol and Capen 1988b). Both low-calcium diet and bisphosphonates decrease hypercalcemia and normalize urinary calcium excretion (Rosol and Capen 1987).

One distinct difference to the human syndrome of HHM is the significantly increased serum level of 1,25-$(OH)_2D$ (Rosol et al. 1986a). Extracts from the tumor line contained bone and kidney adenylate cyclase-stimulating activity, which was inhibited by the PTH antagonist bovine PTH (3–34) amide (Rosol et al. 1987). Tumor extracts and conditioned tissue culture media from CAC-8 significantly increased in vitro bone resorption in neonatal mouse calvaria (Rosol et al. 1986b). This in vitro bone-resorbing activity was not suppressible by indomethacin. The PTH antagonist bovine PTH (3–34) amide did not inhibit the CAC-8-stimulated or bPTH(1–34)-induced bone resorption. But, in 1988, Rosol found that the CAC-8-stimulated bone resorption in vitro is indeed significantly inhibited by higher molar concentrations of the PTH antagonist bPTH(3–34) amide (Rosol and Capen 1988a,b). In 1990 he identified PTHrP using western and northern analysis in the CAC-8 tumor line, demonstrating that PTHrP is probably important in the pathogenesis of humoral hypercalcemia of malignancy (Rosol et al. 1990). However, PTHrP may not be the only responsible cytokine. Merryman and coworkers (1989) showed that the CAC-8 model, in addition to the PTH-like factor, produces TFGα and TGFβ that were separable by reverse phase or cation exchange HPLC. Further studies using this model would be useful to investigate the role of the cosecretion of TGFs and PTHrP in the pathogenesis of HHM.

Transplantation of Human Tumors into Immunodeficient Mice

Several human tumors associated with hypercalcemia have been established in nude mice, a model which allows the testing of human tumors in vivo (see Table 2). Esophageal carcinoma (KEsC-2), pancreatic carcinoma (FA-6), melanoma (SEKI) and lung carcinoma (Lu-65A, Lu-61), all associated with hypercalcemia, cause hypercalcemia in transplanted nude mice. All these tumors have been positive for PTHrP in northern blot analysis (Nagata et al. 1989; Miyake et al. 1991). The pancreatic carcinoma FA-6 has also been shown to produce TGFα and β. The cell line Lu-65 synthesizes and releases large amounts of prostaglandin E_2 (Bockman et al. 1983a). Many experiments have been performed on the transplantion of squamous cell carcinoma in nude mice. The nude mice consequently develop hypercalcemia, cachexia, leukocytosis, hypophosphatemia and increased urinary cAMP excretion (Saito et al. 1981; Abramson et al. 1984; Yoneda et al. 1991). Studies revealed that both increased renal calcium resorption and increased bone resorption contribute significantly to the pathogenesis of HHM in this model (Shipley et al. 1988; Kukrea et al. 1988b). Sato and coworkers (1989a) demonstrated for the squamous cell cancer cell line T3M-1 by northern blot hybridization that T3M-1 cells produce mRNA for PTHrP and granulocyte colony-stimulating factor. Furthermore, primer extension analysis revealed that the cells also produce mRNA for interleukin 1α.

The esophageal carcinoma (EC-GI) is another human tumor transplanted into nude mice. In this model PTHrP and interleukin-1α seem to be responsible for mediating HHM (Sato et al. 1989b), whereas for anaplastic lung cancer (SK-Luci-6) PTHrP and TGFα were shown not to be involved in the pathogenesis of the HHM. In renal carcinoma, hypercalcemia of transplanted nude mice was accompanied by increased 1,25-$(OH)_2D$ levels. Transitional cell carcinoma associated with hypercalcemia and increased bone resorption were shown to have elevated circulating prostaglandin levels (Bringhurst et al. 1986; Nemoto et al. 1988). Another tumor in which TGF and IL-1, rather than PTHrP, seem to be relevant for mediating hypercalcemia is the ascites sarcoma 180 (S180A) in nude mice (Suzuki and Yamada 1991). Although mice suffering from HHM normally show increased 1,25-$(OH)_2D$ levels, there is a report that rhabdomyosarcoma-induced hypercalcemia in mice show unchanged 1,25-$(OH)_2D$ levels (Takeuchi et al. 1982). An overview of responsible humoral mediators is given in Table 3.

Humoral Factors Mediating Hypercalcemia

Parathyroid Hormone-Related Protein (PTHrP)

One way to demonstrate the importance of PTHrP in the pathogenesis of humoral hypercalcemia of malignancy is the infusion of synthetic PTHrP. Rosol et al. (1988) demonstrated that PTHrP mimics the action of native PTH, including elevated 1,25-$(OH)_2D$ levels, when infused into nude mice. Yates et al. (1988) confirmed these results in normal mice. Chinese hamster ovarian (CHO) cells transfected with human PTHrP cDNA also caused hypercalcemia in nude mice (Guise et al. 1992).

PTHrP is the causative factor in the Walker carcinosarcoma (WCS) 256 (Scharla et al. 1991; Torres et al. 1992; de Miguel and Esbrit 1992; Raue et al. 1993). The half-life of PTHrP (53–84) and of PTHrP (1–86) in this model is about 1.5 h (Schilling et al. 1993b), in contrast to the half-life of PTH, which is only a few minutes. PTHrP is also significantly involved in the Leydig cell tumor induced HHM. This was demonstrated by measuring increased circulating immunoreactive PTHrP levels and by immunoneutralization with antiserum against PTHrP (Gaich and Burtis 1990; Henderson et al. 1990).

Table 3. Transplantation of human tumors into athymic mice and the responsible humoral mediators of HHM

Origin	Abbreviation	Responsible factor/s				
		PTHrP	TGFα and β	PGE_2	IL-1α	1,25-$(OH)_2$D
Pancreatic	FA-6	+	+	–	–	–
Esophageal	KEsC-2	+	–	–	–	–
Melanoma	SEKI	+	–	–	–	–
Lung cancer	Lu-65A	+	–	+	–	–
Lung cancer	Lu-61	+	–	–	–	–
Squamous cell CA		+[a]	–	–	+[a]	–
Eosophagus	EC-GI	+	–	–	+	–
Renal carcinoma		(+)	–	–	–	↑
Prostate carcinoma 9479		(+)	–	–	–	↑
Anaplastic lung	SK-Luci-6	n	β, no α	–	–	–
Transitional cell CA	TCC	n[a]	n[a]	+[a]	–	–
Ascites sarcoma 180	S180A	n[a]	+[a]	–	+[a]	–
Rhabdomyosarcoma		–	–	+	–	→

+, is involved in the mediation; (+), is probably involved, definitive proof lacking; n, results suggest that factor is not involved in the mediation of HHM; ↑, elevated circulating levels; →, normal circulating levels; –, has not been tested to date.
[a] Results obtained by in vitro studies (see text).

Western and northern analysis revealed that the canine adenocarcinoma (CAC-8) tissue contains a homologue to human PTHrP that seems likely to be the causative agent in the pathogenesis of humoral hypercalcemia of malignancy. In this animal model, the cosecretion of TGFs may also be a significant factor for the development of HHM (Merryman et al. 1989). PTHrP was also shown to be responsible for mediating hypercalcemia in human tumors transplanted into nude mice. The infusion of antibodies against PTHrP in mice bearing a human squamous cell carcinoma or a human laryngeal carcinoma lowered serum calcium (Kukreja et al. 1988b, 1990). Sato et al. (1993) also found that passive immunization against PTHrP can continuously ameliorate the hypercalcemia and furthermore markedly prolong the survival time of tumor-bearing mice.

Besides its effects on the calcium metabolism, PTHrP has been shown to be a regulator or modulator of cardiovascular function. By infusion of PTH (1–34) and PTHrP (1–34), Nickols and coworkers showed (1989) that PTHrP and PTH decrease blood pressure by relaxing vascular tissue in an endothelium-independent manner and that these peptides directly increase heart rate, contractility and coronary flow. The same results were obtained by Musso et al. (1989), who demonstrated that PTHrP causes vasorelaxation and stimulation of microvascular adenylate cyclase in the isolated rat kidney. Indeed there are two case reports of patients suffering from HHM who developed hypotension and tachycardia (Mundy 1987). In contrast, Leydig cell tumor bearing rats with elevated PTHrP serum levels exhibit hypertension (Sowers and Barrett 1982; Nyby et al. 1987).

There is general agreement that PTHrP and PTH interact with the same receptors in kidney and bone. Although immunologically distinct, PTHrP and PTH have been shown to bind to the same receptor in cultured rat bone cells and canine renal membranes (Juppner et al. 1988; Nissenson et al. 1988). Using rats infused with synthetic PTHrP (1–34), Horiuchi and coworkers (1990) demonstrated that PTH antagonists reverse the PTHrP effects in vivo. In vitro data of Donahue et al. (1990) are generally consistent with PTHrPs acting through the PTH receptor, but differences in the effects of the inhibitory PTH analogs bovine PTH (3–34) and bovine PTH (7–34) on PTH and PTHrP action suggest as yet unexplained complexities, such as the existence of a PTH/PTHrP receptor family.

Transforming Growth Factor (TGF)

Transforming growth factors (TGFs) are defined by their ability to stimulate the formation of colonies in soft agar of certain indicator cell lines (Goustin et al. 1986). TGFs consist of two major subclasses: TGFα and TGFβ. It is known that TGFα binds to the receptor for epidermal growth factor (EGF) and is able to stimulate bone resorption in vitro (Ibbotson et al. 1985b). TGFβ is a completely distinct protein from TGFα and has its own receptor

(Goustin et al. 1986). TGFβ is able to induce proliferation or differentiation of many different cell types and to stimulate bone resorption in vitro (Stern et al. 1985; Mundy et al. 1985; Rosol and Capen 1988b) and in vivo (Yates et al. 1992).

It was shown that TGFβ is secreted by the Leydig cell tumor (Ibbotson et al. 1983, 1985a; Insogna et al. 1987). The importance of this cosecretion of TGFβ with PTHrP by the Leydig cell tumor has not been well studied to date. The evidence that has linked TGFα closely to hypercalcemia is that bone-resorbing activity in the Leydig cell tumor could be completely inhibited by antiserum to the EGF receptor which blocked the effects of TGFα in vitro (Ibbotson et al. 1985a). But Shevrin et al. (1987) demonstrated that EGF infusion into nude mice had no effect on serum and urine calcium values although EGF-infused animals exhibited the known biological effects of significantly greater gastric and pancreatic weights than controls. Thus, the significancy of the cosecretion of TGFs in mediating the syndrome of HHM has not yet been shown in detail.

Both TGFα and TGFβ have been separated in the canine adenocarcinoma model by reverse phase cation exchange HPLC. Again, the role of TGFs as causative agents in this syndrome has not been verified.

Interleukin-1α (IL-1α)

Malignant tumors associated with hypercalcemia may secrete several peptide cytokines, including interleukin-1α (IL-1α) (Sato et al. 1988, 1989b). IL-1α was shown to be able to stimulate bone resorption and to cause hypercalcemia in mice (Sabatini et al. 1988; Lorenzo et al. 1988). Using infusion models in rats, Torring et al. (1992) showed that the combination of IL-1α with PTHrP reduced hypercalcemia. Hypophosphatemia and phosphaturia occur due to strong inhibition of the renal effects of PTHrP. Thus cosecretion of IL-1α with PTHrP may be able to modify the clinical expression of HHM.

Interleukin-6 (IL-6)

The effects of interleukin-6 (IL-6) in vivo were assessed by inoculating CHO cells transfected with the murine IL-6 gene in nude mice. This caused hypercalcemia, leukocytosis and cachexia (Black et al. 1991). These results suggest that increased circulating levels of IL-6 may contribute to the syndrome of HHM.

Yoneda et al. (1993) were able to demonstrate that neutralizing antibodies to human IL-6 lower serum calcium in nude mice carrying a human tumor associated with increased IL-6 production. There was no effect on blood calcium in hypercalcemic nude mice carrying tumors not associated with increased IL-6 production and normocalcemic tumor-bearing nude mice. This suggests that increased production of IL-6 may contribute to disturbances in calcium homeostasis in some malignancies.

1,25-Dihydroxyvitamin D [1,25-(OH)₂D]

There are conflicting data regarding the role of 1,25-$(OH)_2D$ in HHM. In animal models of HHM, or by infusion of PTHrP, elevated levels of 1,25-$(OH)_2D$ are found (Horiuchi et al. 1987; Strewler et al. 1986; Nesbitt and Drezner 1990; Scharla et al. 1989). In humans with HHM, 1,25-$(OH)_2D$ concentrations are generally low (Stewart et al. 1980; Ralston et al. 1984; Yamamoto et al. 1987; Schilling et al. 1993c). Ikeda et al. (1988), using a nude rat model implanted with oral cavity cancer, found all features to be similar to the human HHM syndrome except for markedly elevated serum 1,25-$(OH)_2D$ levels. Thus the regulation of 1,25-$(OH)_2D$ by PTHrP seems to be species dependent.

The duration of elevated PTHrP levels may also be important for the regulation of 1,25-$(OH)_2D$. Fraher et al. (1992) demonstrated that short infusion of synthetic PTHrP(1–34) over 12 h leads to increased serum 1,25-$(OH)_2D$ levels in humans. This is in contrast to suppressed 1,25-$(OH)_2D$ levels in patients suffering from HHM due to "chronically" elevated PTHrP serum levels (Schilling et al. 1993c).

It is conceivable that concomitant tumor secretion of other cytokines blocks the effect of PTHrP on renal synthesis of 1,25-$(OH)_2D$ (Fukumoto et al. 1989). However, considering the analogy between malignancy and primary hyperparathyroidism, levels of 1,25-$(OH)_2D$ are subject to two countervailing influences: the direct effect of PTH or PTHrP to stimulate 1,25-$(OH)_2D$ synthesis is opposed by the effect of increased levels of serum calcium itself to inhibit it. In normal humans and other species, chronic infusion of PTH to produce mild sustained hypercalcemia results in suppression of serum 1,25-$(OH)_2D$ levels (Hulter et al. 1985). This suppression of 1,25-$(OH)_2D$ is the consequence of hypercalcemia: when the serum calcium level is transiently "clamped" in the normal range, serum 1,25-$(OH)_2D$ rises to normal levels, but falls promptly when the "clamp" is discontinued and hypercalcemia recurs (Strewler and Nissenson 1990). In analogy, in patients suffering from HHM, suppressed serum 1,25-$(OH)_2D$ levels rise when serum calcium is decreased by bisphosphonate therapy (Schilling et al. 1993c). Thus it seems possible that low concentrations of 1,25-$(OH)_2D$ in malignancy similarly reflect a suppressive effect of hypercalcemia.

Another regulator of circulating 1,25-$(OH)_2D$ in HHM is serum phosphorus. Kukreja et al. (1989) measured in vitro 25-hydroxyvitamin D_1-hydroxylase (1-OHase) activity in kidneys from athymic mice implanted with a hypercalcemia-producing human lung tumor. They found that low serum phosphorus increased 1-OHase activity and vice versa. Thus, in nude mice, hypophosphatemia is required for expression of enhanced 1-OHase activity leading to increased 1,25-$(OH)_2D$ serum levels.

Prostaglandins

Prostaglandin-mediated hypercalcemia is relatively rare in humans. This is in contrast to some animal models, in which prostaglandins seem to play a significant role. Prostanglandins were thought to be the responsible factor in the VX-2 carcinoma. But, as mentioned above, there are conflicting data showing a doubtful role for prostaglandins in this syndrome.

The $HSDM_1$ fibrosarcoma model in mice is another example of prostaglandin-mediated hypercalcemia (see above). Mitnick et al. (1992) examined the effect of PTHrP on prostaglandin E_2 (PGE_2) secretion in vitro by human osteoblast-like cells. Along with an augmentation of peptide length, varying from 36 to 141 amino acids, a significant increase in efficacy for PGE_2 release was seen. Thus the carboxy-terminal region of PTHrP may partly cause hypercalcemia by release of the potent bone-active cytokine PGE_2.

Tumor Necrosis Factor (TNF)

Elevated levels of TNF have been shown in the Leydig cell tumor model (see above). TNF is known to cause hypercalcemia in vivo. This has been shown using CHO cells transfected with the human TNF gene (Johnson et al. 1989). In nude mice carrying these CHO tumors expressing human TNF, there was also evidence of increased osteoclastic bone resorption. Urinary calcium excretion was also increased whereas urinary cAMP exrection was unchanged.

Using nude mice transplanted with a human squamous cell carcinoma of the maxilla (MH-85), Yonedo et al. showed (1991) that injection of polyclonal neutralizing antibodies raised against murine TNF decreased serum calcium. As already mentioned above, TNF is not produced by the tumor cells but rather by host cells of the macrophage lineage (Yoneda et al. 1991). Thus the paraneoplastic syndrome of HHM may be caused by the production of TNF factors by normal host cells stimulated by the presence of the tumor.

Therapy of HHM

Bisphosphonates

The Walker carcinosarcoma (WCS) 256 has often been used to test bisphosphonates. Guaitani et al. (1984) showed for WCS 256 and other murine tumor models that disodium etidronate is able to reduce hypercalcemia and urinary calcium excretion and to inhibit formation of bone metastases. Besides the inhibition of bone metastases, etidronate does not exert direct antineoplastic activity on the tumor itself (Garattini et al. 1987; Bassani et al. 1990). The bisphosphonate pamidronate (APD) revealed the same effects (Jung et al. 1984; Wingen et al. 1986). WCS rats treated with APD show increased survival (Krempien et al. 1988). Newly developed, more potent bisphosphonates such as BM 21.9055 lead to inhibition of bone resorption, hypercalcemia and urinary calcium excretion without alteration of the renal handling of calcium (Rizzoli et al. 1992).

The inhibition of the formation of bone metastases by bisphosphonates is of great clinical interest. If potential risk groups for bone metastasis can be defined, these groups might profit from prophylactic bisphosphonate treatment to inhibit tumor-induced bone destruction.

Ethiofos (WR-2721)

WR-2721 [S-2-(3aminopropylaminoethyl) phosphorothioic acid] is a radioprotective and chemoprotective compound (Yuhas and Storer 1969; Yuhas et al. 1980) which was found to be an effective hypocalcemic agent through inhibition of PTH secretion (Glover et al. 1983). In addition, Ethiofos shows a further mechanism of hypocalcemic action. It leads to PTH-independent inhibition of osteoclast-mediated bone resorption (Attie et al. 1985). Weiss et al. (1986) confirmed this inhibition of bone resorption using the WCS 256 animal model. A third mechanism, by which WR-2721 lowers serum calcium, is a decrease in renal calcium reabsorption, which was apparent in the Leydig model (Hirschel-Scholz et al. 1986).

Vitamin D

Besides its hypercalcemic effects, the active vitamin D metabolite 1,25-$(OH)_2D$ has antiproliferative properties. These antiproliferative effects were tested in the WCS 256. When the rats were treated from day 0 of tumor transplantation, 1,25-$(OH)_2D$ inhibited the development of the Walker tumor, whereas treatment from day 4 was ineffective in reducing tumor weight (Cohen-Solal et al. 1993). 24R,25-Dihydroxycholecalciferol, another active metabolite of vitamin D, was also shown to have an antimetastatic effect and prolonged survival in mice bearing the hypercalcemia causing Lewis lung carcinoma (Maeda et al. 1988). The influence of 24R,25-dihydroxycholecalciferol on calcium metabolism was not tested. The hypercalcemic effect of 1,25-$(OH)_2D$ will prohibit its therapeutic use in hypercalcemia of malignancy. The therapeutic use of newly developed vitamin D analogues, which have less hypercalcemic and more antiproliferative effects, awaits testing.

Glucocorticoids

Dexamethasone was shown to reduce PTHrP secretion and storage of WCS 256 cells in vitro (Wagner et al. 1993). We could not confirm these results in vivo. Treatment of WCS rats with dexamethasone (1 mg/kg daily) from day 4 after transplantation had no effect on tumor growth or PTHrP secretion (Schilling et al. 1993a).

Aspirin and Indomethacin

In the 1980s Powles et al. (1973) found prevention of osteolytic bone deposits and hypercalcemia in WCS by aspirin and indomethacin, whereas soft tissue tumor deposits were unaffected by these drugs. The possible clinical use of aspirin in inhibition of bone metastases has not been shown to date.

Thionapthene-2-carboxylic Acid (TNCA)

Thionapthene-2-carboxylic acid (TNCA) has been shown to block bone resorption in organ culture and to lower serum calcium concentrations in hypercalcemic rats (Raisz et al. 1985; Johannesson et al. 1985). Decker and coworkers (1989) tested thionapthene-2-carboxylic acid lysine salt (TNLY) for its effects on serum calcium concentration and survival in rats bearing the Leydig cell tumor. They found that the onset of hypercalcemia was prevented without any influence on overall survival.

Acetazolamide

The enzyme carbonic anhydrase has been suggested as a critical participant in osteoclast-mediated bone resorption. It is suggested that when resorption occurs the extracellular space between the osteoclast and the bone surface is acidified (Baron et al. 1985). The carbonic anhydrase is considered to play a major role in acid generation by osteoclasts (Hall and Kenny 1985). Brown and coworkers (1990) examined the effect of the carbonic anhydrase inhibitor acetazolamide on the hypercalcemia induced by the Leydig cell tumor. Acetazolamide lowered the serum calcium without influence on serum phosphorus, urine calcium, urine phosphorus or nephrogenous cyclic AMP excretion. This is in contrast to bisphosphonates, which diminish urinary calcium excretion (Guaitani et al. 1984; Rizzoli et al. 1992). Thus, acetazolamide does not seem to be as potent as bisphosphonates in inhibition of bone resorption.

Mithramycin (MMC)

Mithramycin was tested in the transplantable canine adenocarcinoma in nude mice. Mithramycin decreased serum calcium concentration and urine calcium excretion to the range of control non-tumor-bearing mice at day 5 after a single injection (8 mg/kg) in CAC-8 tumor-bearing mice. Osteoclasts from CAC-8-bearing nude mice after mithramycin administration were decreased in size and had small ruffled borders. In vitro, bone resorption induced by CAC-8 extract was reduced by mithramycin (Rosol and Capen 1987). Similar results were obtained in the canine perianal gland carcinoma (CAC-9), in which mithramycin decreased serum calcium and the tumor volume 2 weeks postinjection (Nishikawa et al. 1986). Rosol et al. (1992a) administered mithramycin (0.1 mg/kg) at days 0 and 7 to eight beagle dogs. They found that mithramycin inhibits osteoclastic bone resorption and decreases serum calcium.

Interleukin-4 (IL-4)

Interleukin (IL-4) is known to inhibit bone resorption stimulated by systemic and local factors such as parathyroid hormone-related protein (PTHrP), parathyroid hormone (PTH), 1,25-$(OH)_2D$, IL-1α, IL-1β and prostaglandin E_2 in vitro (Watanabe et al. 1990). Nagasaki and coworkers (1991) tested the hypocalcemic effect of IL-4 infusion by minipumps in mice. IL-4 inhibited plasma calcium elevation induced by PTHrP(1–34) infusion in mice and prevented HHM in nude mice bearing a squamous cell lung carcinoma (Lu-61) or a giant cell lung carcinoma (Lu-65A).

Murine γ-Interferon

Murine γ-interferon is a potent inhibitor of bone resorption in vitro (Peterlik et al. 1985; Gowen et al. 1986). This inhibition of bone resorption in vitro was tested in vivo using the EC-GI-bearing nude mice. Sato and coworkers (1992) found a prolonged decrease of serum calcium and urinary calcium excretion after injection of murine γ-interferon. Human γ-interferon was completely ineffective.

cis-*Platinum (DDP)*

The cytotoxic agent *cis*-platinum (DDP) was tested by Kukla et al. (1984) in athymic mice bearing a human squamous cell lung carcinoma. They found a significant reduction in serum calcium in hypercalcemic tumor-bearing mice compared to normal saline-treated mice. Lad and coworkers (1987) used DDP successfully as treatment for HHM in patients. The hypocalcemic effect of DDP may be due to inhibition of bone resorption, as DDP was shown to diminish the number of osteoclasts and to inhibit bone resorption in vitro in the neonatal mouse calvarial bone resorption assay (Abramson et al. 1988).

Calcium Channel Antagonists

The calcium channel antagonists (CAAs) amlodipine, diltiazem and verapamil were tested in nude mice trasplanted with a human breast cancer cell line. The CAAs inhibited HT-39 human breast cancer cell proliferation in a concentration-dependent manner in vitro (Taylor and Simpson 1992). The same results were obtained in vivo, where the CAAs acted to blunt breast tumor progression in nude mice. The influence of CAAs on hypercalcemia was not tested. As known from clinical trials, the long-term use of these drugs, at the concentrations used in the mice experiment, in the treatment of hypertension is not associated with significant toxicities. Thus CAAs may have specific actions to inhibit cancer cell growth in vivo, with no observed side effects.

Gallium Nitrate

Gallium nitrate (GaN) is the anhydrate of the naturally occurring heavy metal. In the 1980s gallium-67 was used for tumor imaging (Winchell et al. 1970). GaN has demonstrated antitumor activity in a variety of murine models, including the Walker carcinosarcoma 256, fibrosarcoma M-89, adenocarcinoma 755, mammary carcinoma YMC, reticulum cell carcinoma A-RCS, lymphoma P1798, leukemia K-1964, and osteosarcoma 124F (Foster et al. 1986). GaN was shown to inhibit calcium resorption from bone in vitro (Bockman et al. 1983b; Hall and Chambers 1990) and to be an effective treatment for cancer-related hypercalcemia in humans (Warrell et al. 1984). The mechanism of the hypocalcemic effect of GaN is unclear. Cournot-Witmer and coworkers (1987) found, using normal rats, that GaN does not inhibit the activity of osteoblasts in rats and does not interfere with mineralization but increases the number of osteoclasts through stimulation of parathyroid gland activity, induced by a fall in serum calcium. The hypocalcemic effect of GaN seems to be related to skeletal resistance to PTH and to increased renal calcium loss. These in vivo data are contradictory to recently published in vitro data by Ridefelt et al. (1992), who found that gallium inhibits PTH release of the parathyroid cells.

Passive Immunization

As described above, the infusion of antibodies against possible mediators of hypercalcemia such as PTHrP (Kukreja et al. 1988b, 1990; Henderson et al. 1990; Sato et al. 1993) and IL-6 (Yoneda et al. 1993) was shown to lead to a normalization of hypercalcemia in tumor-bearing murine animals. Furthermore it was shown that antibodies against PTHrP markedly prolong survival time of hypercalcemic nude mice (Sato et al. 1993). Thus, if a monoclonal antibody against PTHrP could be synthesized, then passive immunization against PTHrP would be a specific and potent treatment for patients with HHM.

References

Abramson EC, Kukla LJ, Shevrin DH, Lad TE, McGuire WP, Kukreja SC (1984) A model for malignancy-associated humoral hypercalcemia. Calcif Tissue Int 36(5): 563–567

Abramson EC, Chang J, Mayer M, Kukla LJ, Shevrin DH, Lad TE, Buschman R, Kukreja SC (1988) Effects of cisplatin on parathyroid hormone- and human lung tumor-induced bone resorption. J Bone Miner Res 3(5):541–546

Alam I, Voelkel EF, Tashjian AH Jr, Levine L (1980) Analysis by high performance liquid chromatography of cyclooxygenase products of arachidonic acid metabolism in plasma of rabbits bearing the VX2 carcinoma. Prostaglandins Med 4(4): 227–237

Anger B, Bockman R, Andreeff M, Erlandson R, Jhanwar S, Kameya T, Saigo P, Wright W, Beattie EJ Jr, Oettgen HF, Old LJ (1982) Characterization of two newly established human cell lines from patients with large-cell anaplastic lung carcinoma. Cancer 50(8):1518–1529

Attie M, Fallon MD, Spar B, Wolf JS, Slatopolsky E, Goldfarb S (1985) Bone and parathyroid inhibitory effects of S-2(3-aminopropylamino) ethylphosphorothioic acid. J Clin Invest 75:1191–1197

Baron R, Neff L, Louvard D, Courtoy P (1985) Cell-mediated extracellular acidification and bone resorption: evidence for a low pH in resorbing lacunae and localization of a 100-kD lysosomal membrane protein at the osteoclast ruffled border. J Cell Biol 101:2210–2222

Barrett CP, Cubitt JG, Donati EJ (1978) Elevated serum calcium concentrations in mammary tumor bearing C3H/Fg mice without any metastases. Lab Anim Sci 18:34–37

Bassani D, Sabatini M, Scanziani E, Francesco L, Coccioli G, Guaitani A, Bartosek I (1990) Bone invasion by Walker 256 carcinoma, line A in young and adult rats: effects of etidronate. Oncology 47:160–165

Berger ME, Golub MS, Sowers JR, Brickman AS, Nyby M, Troyer H, Rude RK, Singer FR, Horrst R, Deftos LJ (1982) Hypercalcemia in association with a Leydig cell tumor in the rat: a model for tumor-induced hypercalcemia in man. Life Sci 30(18):1509–1515

Black K, Garrett IR, Mundy GR (1991) Chinese hamster ovarian cells transfected with the murine interleukin-6 gene cause hypercalcemia as well as cachexia, leukocytosis and thrombocytosis in tumor-bearing nude mice. Endocrinology 128(5):2657–2659

Bockman RS, Bellin A, Repo MA, Hickok NJ, Kameya T (1983a) In vivo and in vitro biological activities of two human cell lines derived from anaplastic lung cancers. Cancer Res 43(9):4511–4516
Bockman RS, Repo MA, Warrell RP Jr (1983b) Inhibition of in vitro bone resorption by gallium nitrate (abstract). Calcif Tissue Int 35:637
Bringhurst FR, Bierer BE, Godeau F, Neyhard N, Varner V, Segre GV (1986) Humoral hypercalcemia of malignancy. Release of a prostaglandin-stimulating bone-resorbing factor in vitro by human transitional-cell carcinoma cells. J Clin Invest 77(2):456–464
Brown GM, Morris CA, Mitnick MA, Insogna KL (1990) Treatment of humoral hypercalcemia of malignancy in rats with inhibitors of carbonic anhydrase. J Bone Miner Res 5(10):1037–1041
Burtis WJ, Insogna KL, Broadus AE, Stewart AF (1986) Two species of adenylate cyclase-stimulating activity in the murine squamous carcinoma model of humoral hypercalcemia of malignancy. Endocrinology 118:1982–1988
Chew DJ, Carothers M (1989) Hypercalcemia. Vet Clin North Am Small Anim Pract 19(2):265–287
Cohen-Solal M, Bouizar Z, Denne MA, Graulet AM, Guéris A, de Vernejoul J, de Vernejoul MC (1993) Low doses of 1,25-$(OH)_2D_3$ dramatically inhibit the in vivo development of the Walker carcinoma in rats. J Bone Miner Res 7[Suppl 1]:245
Cournot-Witmer G, Bourdeau A, Lieberherr M, Thil CL, Plachot JJ, Enault G, Bourdon R, Balsan S (1987) Bone modeling in gallium nitrate-treated rats. Calcif Tissue Int 40:270–275
Coyle P, Rofe AM, Bourgeois CS, Conyers RA (1990) Biochemical manifestations of a rat mammary adenocarcinoma-producing cachexia: in vivo and in vitro studies. Immunol Cell Biol 68(3):147–153
Decker JE, Morrison NE, Lorenzo JA, Samour CM, McCarron BA, Raisz LG (1989) The effects of thionaphthene-2-carboxylic acid-lysine on the hypercalcemia of malignancy in the rat. Calcif Tissue Int 44:61–64
Delmonte L, Liebelt AG, Liebelt RA (1966) Granulopoiesis and thrombopoiesis in mice bearing transplanted mammary cancer. Cancer Res 26:149–159
De Miguel F, Esbrit P (1992) Isolation of a 18000-Da molecular weight form of parathyroid hormone-related protein from the rat Walker carcinosarcoma 256. Cancer Lett 66:201–206
Donahue HJ, Fryer MJ, Heath H III (1990) Structure-function relationships for full-length recombinant parathyroid hormone-related peptide and its amino-terminal fragments: effects on cytosolic calcium ion mobilization and adenylate cyclase activation in rat osteoblast-like cells. Endocrinology 126(3):1471–1477
Doppelt SH, Slovik DM, Neer RM, Nolan J, Zusman RM, Potts JT Jr (1982) Gut mediated hypercalcemia in rabbits bearing VX2 carcinoma: new mechanism for tumor induced hypercalcemia. Proc Natl Acad Sci USA 79:640–644
D'Souza SM, Ibbotson KJ, Mundy GR (1984a) Gallium nitrate inhibits calcium resorption from bone and is effective treatment for cancer-related hypercalcemia. J Clin Invest 73(5):1487–1490
D'Souza SM, Ibbotson KJ, Smith DD, Mundy GR (1984b) Production of a macromolecular bone-resorbing factor by the hypercalcemic variant of the walker rat carcinosarcoma. Endocrinology 115(5):1746–1752
D'Souza SM, Ibbotson KJ, Mundy GR (1984c) Failure of parathyroid hormone antagonists to inhibit in vitro bone resorbing activity produced by two animal models of the humoral hypercalcemia of malignancy. J Clin Invest 74(3): 1104–1107
Engelman RW, Tyler RD, Good RA, Day NK (1985) Hypercalcemia in cats with feline-leukemia-virus-associated leukemia-lymphoma. Cancer 56(4):777–781

Foster BJ, Clagett-Carr K, Hoth D, Leyland-Jones B (1986) Gallium nitrate: the second metal with clinical activity. Cancer Treat Rep 70:1311–1319

Fraher LJ, Hodsman AB, Jonas K, Saunders D, Rose CI, Henderson JE, Hendy GN, Goltzman D (1992) A comparison of the in vivo biochemical responses to exogenous parathyroid hormone-(1–34) [PTH-(1–34)] and PTH-related peptide-(1–34) in man. J Clin Endocrinol Metab 75:417–423

Fukumoto S, Matsumoto T, Yamoto H, Kwahima H, Ueyama Y (1989) Suppression of 1,25-dihydroxyvitamin D in humoral hypercalcemia of malignancy is caused by elaboration of a factor that inhibits renal 1,25-dihydroxyvitamin D production. Endocrinology 124:2057–2062

Gaich G, Burtis WJ (1990) Measurement of circulating parathyroid hormone-related protein in rats with humoral hypercalcemia of malignancy using a two-site immunoradiometric assay. Endocrinology 127(3):1444–1449

Garattini S, Guaitani A, Mantovani A (1987) Effect of etidronate disodium on the interactions between malignancy and bone. Am J Med 82(2A):29–33

Gkonos PJ, Hayes T, Burtis W, Jacoby R, McGuire J, Baron R, Stewart AF (1984) Squamous carcinoma model of humoral hypercalcemia of malignancy. Endocrinology 115(6):2384–2390

Glover DJ, Riley L, Carmichael K, Spar B, Glick J, Agus Z, Slatopolsky E, Attie M, Goldfarb S (1983) Hypocalcemia and inhibition of parathyroid hormone secretion following administration of WR 2721 (a radio- and chemoprotective agent). N Engl J Med 309:1137–1141

Goldhaber P (1960) Enhancement of bone resorption in tissue culture by mouse fibrosarcoma. Proc Am Assoc Cancer Res 3:113

Goustin AS, Leof EB, Shipley GD, Moses HL (1986) Growth factors and cancer. Cancer Res 46:1015–1029

Gowen M, Nedwin GE, Mundy GR (1986) Preferential inhibition of cytokine-stimulated bone resorption by recombinant interferon gamma. J Bone Miner Res 1:469–474

Guaitani A, Polentarutti N, Filippeschi S, Marmonti L, Corti F, Italia C, Coccioli G, Donelli MG, Mantovani A, Garattini S (1984) Effects of disodium etidronate in murine tumor models. Eur J Cancer Clin Oncol 20(5):685–693

Guaitani A, Sabatini M, Coccioli G, Cristina S, Garattini S, Bartosek I (1985) An experimental rat model of local bone cancer invasion and its responsiveness to ethane-1-hydroxy-1,1-bis(phosphonate). Cancer Res 45(5):2206–2209

Guise TA, Chirgwin JM, Favarato G, Boyce BF, Mundy GR (1992) Chinese hamster ovarian cells transfected with human parathyroid hormone-related protein cDNA cause hypercalcemia in nude mice. Lab Invest 67(4):477–485

Gullino PM, Pettigrew HM, Grantham FH (1975) *N*-nitrosomethylurea as mammary gland carcinogen in rats. J Natl Cancer Inst 54(2):401–414

Hall G, Kenny A (1985) Role of carbonic anhydrase in bone resorption induced by 1,25-dihydroxyvitamin D_3 in vitro. Calcif Tissue Int 37:134–142

Hall TJ, Chambers TJ (1990) Gallium inhibits bone resorption by a direct effect on osteoclasts. Bone and Mineral 8:211–216

Heath H III, Weller RE, Mundy GR (1980) Canine lymphosarcoma: a model for study of the hypercalcemia of cancer. Calcif Tissue Int 30:127–133

Henderson J, Bernier S, D'Amour P, Goltzman D (1990) Effects of passive immunization against parathyroid hormone (PTH)-like peptide and PTH in hypercalcemic tumor-bearing rats and normocalcemic controls. Endocrinology 127: 1310–1318

Hilgard P, Schmitt W, Minne H, Ziegler R (1970) Acute hypercalcemia due to Walker carcinosarcoma 256 in the rat. Horm Metab Res 2:253–256

Hirschel-Scholz S, Caverzasio J, Rizzoli R, Bonjour JP (1986) Normalization of hypercalcemia associated with a decrease in renal calcium reabsorption in

Leydig cell tumor-bearing rats treated with WR-2721. J Clin Invest 78(1):319–322

Horiuchi N, Caulfield MP, Fisher JE, Goldman M, McKnee RL, Reagan JE, Levy JJ, Nutt RF, Rodan SB, Schofield TL et al. (1987) Similarity of synthetic peptide from human tumor to parathyroid hormone in vivo and in vitro. Science 38:1566–1568

Horiuchi N, Hongo T, Clemens TL (1990) The synthetic human parathyroid hormone-related protein is inhibited by a parathyroid hormone antagonist in rats in vivo. J Bone Miner Res 5(6):541–545

Hough A Jr, Seyberth H, Oates J, Hartmann W (1977) Changes in bone and bone marrow of rabbits bearing the VX-2 carcinoma. A comparison of local and distant effects. Am J Pathol 87(3):537–552

Hulter HN, Nalloran BP, Toto RD, Peterson JC (1985) Long-term control of plasma calcitriol concentration in dogs and humans: dominant role of plasma calcium concentration in dogs and humans: dominant role of plasma calcium concentration in experimental hyperparathyroidism. J Clin Invest 76:695–702

Hurtado J, Esbrit P, Rapado A (1988) Evidence for an altered tubular handling of calcium in Walker 256 tumour-bearing rats. Med Sci Res 16:571–572

Hurtado J, Esbrit P, Rapado A (1991) Relative role of bone and kidney in the hypercalcaemia associated with the rat Walker carcinosarcoma 256. Eur J Cancer 27(1):76–79

Ibbotson KJ, D'Souza SM, Ng KW, Osborne CK, Niall M, Martin TJ, Mundy GR (1983) Tumor-derived growth factor increases bone resorption in a tumor associated with humoral hypercalcemia of malignancy. Science 1983 Sep 23; 221(4617):1292–1294

Ibbotson KJ, D'Souza SM, Smith DD, Carpenter G, Mundy GR (1985a) EGF receptor antiserum inhibits bone resorbing activity produced by a rat Leydig cell tumor associated with the humoral hypercalcemia of malignancy. Endocrinology 116(1):469–471

Ibbotson KJ, Twardzik DR, Hargreaves WR, Mundy GR (1985b) Stimulation of bone resorption in vitro by synthetic transforming growth factor-alpha. Science 228:1007–1009

Ikeda K, Matsumoto T, Fukumoto S, Kurokawa K, Ueyama Y, Fujishige K, Tamaoki N, Saito T, Ohtake K, Ogata E (1988) A hypercalcemic nude rat model that completely mimics human syndrome of humoral hypercalcemia of malignancy. Calcif Tissue Int 43(2):97–102

Insogna KL, Stewart AF, Vignery AM, Weir EC, Namnum PA, Baron RE, Kirkwood JM, Deftos LM, Broadus AE (1984) Biochemical and histomorphometric characterization of a rat model for humoral hypercalcemia of malignancy. Endocrinology 114(3):888–896

Insogna KL, Weir EC, Wu TL, Stewart AF, Broadus AE, Burtis WJ, Centrella M (1987) Copurification of transforming growth factor beta-like activity with PTH-like and bone-resorbing activities from a tumor associated with humoral hypercalcemia of malignancy. Endocrinology 120(5):2183–2185

Johannesson AJ, Onkelinx C, Rodan GA, Raisz LG (1985) Thionaphtene-2-carboxylic acid: a new antihypercalcemic agent. Endocrinology 117:1508–1511

Johnson RA, Boyce BF, Mundy GR, Roodman GD (1989) Tumors producing human tumor necrosis factor induced hypercalcemia and osteoclastic bone resorption in nude mice. Endocrinology 124(3):1424–1427

Jung A, Bornand J, Mermillod B, Edouard C, Meunier PJ (1984) Inhibition by diphosphonates of bone resorption induced by the Walker tumor of the rat. Cancer Res 44:3007–3011

Juppner H, Abou Samra AB, Uneno S, Gu WX, Potts JT Jr, Segre GV (1988) The parathyroid hormone-like peptide associated with humoral hypercalcemia of

malignancy and parathyroid hormone bind to the same receptor on the plasma membrane of ROS 17/2.8 cells. J Biol Chem 263(18):8557–8560
Kidd JG, Rous P (1940) A transplantable rabbit carcinoma originating in a virus-induced papilloma and containing the virus in masked or altered form. J Exp Med 71:813–838
Klausner JS, Bell FW, Hayden DW, Hegstad RL, Johnston SD (1990) Hypercalcemia in two cats with squamous cell carcinomas. J Am Vet Med Assoc 196(1):103–105
Klein RF, Strewler GJ, Leung SC, Nissenson RA (1987) Parathyroid hormone-like adenylate cyclase-stimulating activity from a human carcinoma is associated with bone-resorbing activity. Endocrinology 120(2):504–511
Krempien B, Wingen F, Eichmann T, Muller M, Schmahl D (1988) Protective effects of a prophylactic treatment with the bisphosphonate 3-amino-1-hydroxy-propane-1,1-bisphosphonic acid on the development of tumor osteopathies in the rat: experimental studies with the Walker carcinosarcoma 256. Oncology 45(1): 41–46
Kukla LJ, Abramson EC, McGuire WP, Shevrin DH, Lad T, Kukreja SC (1984) Cis-platinum treatment for malignancy-associated humoral hypercalcemia in an athymic mouse model. Calcif Tissue Int 36(5):559–562
Kukreja SC, Rosol TJ, Shevrin DH, York PA (1988a) Quantitative bone histo-morphometry in nude mice bearing a human squamous cell lung cancer. J Bone Miner Res 3(3):341–346
Kukreja SC, Shevrin DH, Wimbiscus SA, Ebeling PR, Danks JA, Rodda CP, Wood WI, Martin TJ (1988b) Antibodies to parathyroid hormone-related protein lower serum calcium in athymic mouse models of malignancy-associated hypercalcemia due to human tumors. J Clin Invest 82(5):1798–1802
Kukreja SC, York PA, Nalbantian Brandt C, Shevrin DH, Favus MJ (1989) Effect of hypercalcemia-producing tumor on $1{,}25(OH)_2D_3$ biosynthesis in athymic mice. Am J Physiol 256(2/1):E309–314
Kukreja SC, Rosol TJ, Wimbiscus SA, Shevrin DH, Grill V, Barengolts EI, Martin TJ (1990) Tumor resection and antibodies to parathyroid hormone-related protein cause similar changes on bone histomorphometry in hypercalcemia of cancer. Endocrinology 127(1):305–310
Lad TE, Mishoulam HM, Shevrin DH, Kukla LJ, Abramson EC, Kukreja SC (1987) Treatment of cancer-associated hypercalcemia with cis-platinum. Arch Intern Med 147:329–332
Lau K, Lee M (1983) Mouse CE mammary carcinoma induced hypercalcemia. Calcif Tissue Int 35:660–665
Lee MY, Baylink DJ (1983) Hypercalcemia, excessive bone resorption, and neutro-philia in mice bearing a mammary carcinoma. Proc Soc Exp Biol Med 172(4): 424–429
Lee MY, Liu CC, Lottsfeldt JL, Judkins SA, Howard GA (1987) Production of granulocyte-stimulating and bone cell-modulating activities from a neutrophilia hypercalcemia-inducing murine mammary cancer cell line. Cancer Res 47: 4059–4065
Lee MY, Kaushansky K, Judkins SA, Lottsfeldt JL, Waheed A, Shadduck RK (1989) Mechanisms of tumor-induced neutrophilia: constitutive production of colony-stimulating factors and their synergistic actions. Blood 74(1):115–122
Levine L, Hinkle P, Voelkel E, Tashjian AH Jr (1972) Prostaglandin production by mouse fibrosarcoma cell in culture: inhibition by indomethacin and aspirin. Biochem Biophys Res Commun 47:888–896
Linehan WM, Kish ML, Chen SL, Andriole GL, Santora AC (1986) Human prostate carcinoma causes hypercalcemia in athymic nude mice and produces a factor with parathyroid hormone-like bioactivity. J Urol 135(3):616–620

Linkhart TA, Mohan S, Jennings JC, Baylink DJ (1989) Copurification of osteolytic and transforming growth factor beta activites produced by human lung tumor cells associated with humoral hypercalcemia of malignancy. Cancer Res 49(2):271–278
Lorenzo JA, Sousa SL, Centrella M (1988) Interleukin-1 in combination with transforming growth factor-α produces enhanced bone resorption in vitro. Endocrinology 123:2194–2200
Maeda Y, Yamato H, Hirai T, Kobori N, Fujii T, Kobayashi Y, Saitoh K, Inoguchi E, Hakozaki M, Iijima H et al. (1988) Antitumor and other effects of 24R, 25-dihydroxycholecalciferol in Lewis lung carcinoma causing abnormal calcium metabolism in tumor-bearing mice. Oncology 45:202–205
McCoy DJ, Beasley R (1986) Hypercalcemia associated with malignancy in a horse. J Am Vet Med Assoc 189(1):87–89
Merryman JI, Rosol TJ, Brooks CL, Capen CC (1989) Separation of parathyroid hormone-like activity from transforming growth factor-alpha and -beta in the canine adenocarcinoma (CAC-8) model of humoral hypercalcemia of malignancy. Endocrinology 124(5):2456–2463
Meuten DJ, Cooper BJ, Capen CC, Chew DJ, Kociba GJ (1981) Hypercalcemia associated with an adenocarcinoma derived from the apocrine glands of the anal sac. Vet Pathol 18:454–471
Meuten DJ, Capen CC, Kociba GJ, Chew DJ, Cooper BJ (1982a) Ultrastructural evaluation of adenocarcinomas derived from apocrine glands of the anal sac associated with hypercalcemia in dogs. Am J Pathol 107:167–175
Meuten DJ, Capen CC, Kociba GJ, Cooper BJ (1982b) Hypercalcemia of malignancy: hypercalcemia associated with an adenocarcinoma of the apocrine glands of the anal sac. Am J Pathol 108:366–370
Meuten DJ, Segre GV, Capen CC, Kociba GJ, Voelkel EF, Levine L, Tashjian AH, Chew DJ, Nagode LA (1983a) Hypercalcemia in dogs with adenocarcinoma derived from apocrine glands of the anal sac: biochemical and histomorphometric investigations. Lab Invest 48(4):428–435
Meuten DJ, Kociba GJ, Capen CC, Chew DJ, Segre GV, Levine L, Tashjian AH, Voelkel EF, Nagode LA (1983b) Hypercalcemia in dogs with lymphosarcoma: biochemical, ultrastructural, and histomorphometric investigations. Lab Invest 49(5):553–562
Minne H, Raue F, Bellwinkel S, Ziegler R (1975) The hypercalcaemic syndrome in rats bearing the Walker carcinosarcoma 256. Acta Endocrinol (Copenh) 78(3):613–624
Mitnick M, Isales C, Paliwal I, Insogna K (1992) Parathyroid hormone-related protein stimulates prostaglandin E2 release from human osteoblast-like cells: modulating effect of peptide length. J Bone Miner Res 7(8):887–896
Miyake Y, Yamaguchi K, Honda S, Nagasaki K, Tsuchihashi T, Mori M, Kimura S, Abe K (1991) Production of parathyroid hormone-related protein in tumour xenografts in nude mice presenting with hypercalcaemia. Br J Cancer 63(2): 252–256
Mundy GR (1987) The hypercalcemia of malignancy. Kidney Int 31:142–155
Mundy GR (1991) Ectopic production of calciotropic peptides. Endocrinol Metab Clin North Am 20(3):473–487
Mundy GR, Ibbotson KJ, D'Souza SM (1985) Tumor products and the hypercalcemia of malignancy. J Clin Invest 82:1–6
Musso MJ, Plante M, Judes C, Barthelmebs M, Helwig JJ (1989) Renal vasodilatation and microvessel adenylate cyclase stimulation by synthetic parathyroid hormone-like protein fragments. Eur J Pharmacol 174:139–151
Nagasaki K, Yamaguchi K, Miyake Y, Hayashi C, Honda S, Urakami K, Miki K, Kimura S, Watanabe T, Abe K (1989) In vitro and in vivo antagonists against

parathyroid hormone-related protein. Biochem Biophys Res Commun 158(3): 1036–1042

Nagasaki K, Yamaguchi K, Watanabe K, Eto S, Abe K (1991) Interleukin-4 blocks parathyroid hormone-related protein-induced hypercalcemia in vivo. Biochem Biophys Res Commun 178(2):694–698

Nagata N, Akatsu T, Kugai N, Yasutomo Y, Kinoshita T, Kosano H, Shimauchi T, Takatani O, Ueyama Y (1989) The tumor cells (FA-6) established from a pancreatic cancer associated with humoral hypercalcemia of malignancy: a simultaneous production of parathyroid hormone-like activity and transforming growth factor activity. Endocrinol Jpn 36(1):75–85

Nemoto R, Uchida K, Tsutsumi M, Koiso K, Satoh T (1988) Bone resorption induced by transplanted bladder tumor (MBT-2) in mice. J Urol 139(3):650–652

Nesbitt T, Drezner MK (1990) Abnormal parathyroid hormone-related peptide stimulation of renal 25-hydroxyvitamin d-1-hydroxylase in hyp mice: evidence for a generalized defect of enzyme activity in the proximal convoluted tubule. Endocrinology 127:843–848

Nickols GA, Nana AD, Nickols MA, DiPette DJ, Asimakis GK (1989) Hypotension and cardiac stimulation due to the parathyroid hormone-related protein, humoral hypercalcemia of malignancy factor. Endocrinology 125(2):834–841

Nishikawa S, Rosol TJ, Capen CC (1986) Effects of mithramycin on transplantable canine perianal gland carcinoma (CAC-9) in nude mice: biochemical, histomorphometric, and ultrastructural investigations. Vet Pathol 23(6):698–705

Nissenson RA, Diep D, Strewler GJ (1988) Synthetic peptides comprising the amino-terminal sequence of a parathyroid hormone-like protein from human malignancies. J Biol Chem 263:12866–12871

Norrdin RW, Powers BE (1983) Bone changes in hypercalcemia of malignancy in dogs. J Am Vet Med Assoc 183(4):441–444

Nyby MD, Berger ME, Golub MS, Brickman AS (1987) Decreased vascular reactivity to norepinephrine in Fischer rats with neoplasia-induced hypercalcemia. Life Sci 40(14):1397–1404

Orr FW, Millar-Book W, Singh G (1990) Chemotactic activity of bone and platelet-derived TGF-β for bone-metastasizing rat Walker 256 carcinosarcoma cells. Invasion Metastasis 10:241–252

Patnaik AK, MacEwen EG, Erlandson RA, Lieberman PH, Liu SK (1978) Mediastinal parathyroid adenocarcinoma in a dog. Vet Pathol 15:55–63

Peterlik M, Hoffmann O, Swetly P, Kraushofer K, Koller K (1985) Recombinant γ-interferon inhibits prostaglandin-mediated and parathyroid hormone-induce bone resorption in cultured neonatal mouse calvaria. FEBS Lett 188:287–290

Powles TJ, Clark SA, Easty DM, Easty GC, Neville AM (1973) The inhibition by aspirin and indomethacin of osteolytic tumor deposits and hypercalcaemia in rats with Walker tumour, and its possible application to human breast cancer. Br J Cancer 28(4):316–321

Raisz LG, Alander C, Onkelinx C, Rodan GA (1985) Effects of thionapthene-2-carboxylic acid and related compounds on bone resorption in organ culture. Calcif Tissue Int 37:556–559

Ralston SH, Cowan RA, Robertson Ag, Gardner MD, Boyle IT (1984) Circulating vitamin D metabolites and hypercalcemia of malignancy. Acta Endocrinol (Copenh) 106:556–563

Raue F, Schilling T, Blind E, Baier R, Ziegler R (1993) PTH-related protein is the responsible factor for the syndrome of humoral hypercalcemia of malignancy in the Walker carcinosarcoma 256 rat model. Endocrine Society, 75th annual meeting, Las Vegas, Nevada, p 1415

Rice BF, Ponthier R, Miller M (1971) Hypercalcemia and neoplasia: a model system. Endocrinology 88:1210–1216

Rice BF, Roth LM, Cole FE, MacPhee AA, Davis K, Ponthier R, Sternberg WH (1975) Hypercalcemia and neoplasia: biologic, biochemical, and ultrastructural studies of a hypercalcemia-producing Leydig cell tumor of the rat. Lab Invest 33(4):428–439

Riddle CV, Lee MY, Lee MJ (1987) Morphological characterization of a granulocytosis/hypercalcemia-inducing murine mammary carcinoma cell line. Anat Rec 219(2):127–134

Ridefelt P, Heilman P, Ljunggren Ö, Ljunghail S, Akerström G, Rastad J, Gylfe E (1992) Ga^{3+} inhibits parathyroid hormone release without interacting with the Ca^{2+} receptor of the parathyroid cell. Biochem Biophys Res Comm 186(1): 556–561

Rizzoli R, Caverzasio J, Fleisch H, Bonjour JP (1986) Parathyroid hormone-like changes in renal calcium and phosphate reabsorption induced by Leydig cell tumor in thyroparathyroidectomized rats. Endocrinology 119(3):1004–1009

Rizzoli R, Caverzasion J, Bauss B, Bonjour JP (1992) Inhibition of bone resorption by the bisphosphonate BM 21.9055 is not associated with an alteration of the renal handling of calcium in rats infused with parathyroid hormone-related protein. Bone 13:321–325

Rodan SB, Insogna KL, Vignery AM, Stewart AF, Broadus AE, D'Souza SM, Bertolini DR, Mundy GR, Rodan GA (1983) Factors associated with humoral hypercalcemia of malignancy stimulate adenylate cyclase in osteoblastic cells. J Clin Invest 72(4):1511–1515

Rosol TJ, Capen CC (1987) The effect of low calcium diet, mithramycin, and dichlorodimethylene bisphosphonate on humoral hypercalcemia of malignancy in nude mice transplanted with the canine adenocarcinoma tumor line (CAC-8). J Bone Miner Res 2(5):395–405

Rosol TJ, Capen CC (1988a) Inhibition of in vitro bone resorption by a parathyroid hormone receptor antagonist in the canine adenocarcinoma model of humoral hypercalcemia of malignancy. Endocrinology 122(5):2098–2102

Rosol TJ, Capen CC (1988b) Pathogenesis of humoral hypercalcemia of malignancy. Domest Anim Endocrinol 5(1):1–21

Rosol TJ, Capen CC, Weisbrode SE, Horst RL (1986a) Humoral hypercalcemia of malignancy in nude mouse model of a canine adenocarcinoma derived from apocrine glands of the anal sac. Biochemical, histomorphometric, and ultrastructural studies. Lab Invest 54(6):679–688

Rosol TJ, Capen CC, Minkin C (1986b) In vitro bone resorption activity produced by a hypercalcemic adenocarcinoma tumor line (CAC-8) in nude mice. Calcif Tissue Int 39(5):334–341

Rosol TJ, Capen CC, Brooks CL (1987) Bone and kidney adenylate cyclase-stimulating activity produced by a hypercalcemic canine adenocarcinoma line (CAC-8) maintained in nude mice. Cancer Res 47(3):690–695

Rosol TJ, Capen CC, Horst RL (1988) Effects of infusion of human parathyroid hormone-related protein-(1–40) in nude mice: histomorphometric and biochemical investigations. J Bone Miner Res 3(6):699–706

Rosol TJ, Capen CC, Danks JA, Suva LJ, Steinmeyer CL, Hayman J, Ebeling PR, Martin TJ (1990) Identification of parathyroid hormone-related protein in canine apocrine adenocarcinoma of the anal sac. Vet Pathol 27(2):89–95

Rosol TJ, Chew DJ, Couto CG, Ayl RD, Nagode LA, Capen CC (1992a) Effects of mithramycin on calcium metabolism and bone in dogs. Vet Pathol 29(3):223–229

Rosol TJ, Nagode LA, Couto CG, Hammer AS, Chew DJ, Peterson JL, Ayl RD, Steinmeyer CL, Capen CC (1992b) Parathyroid hormone (PTH)-related protein, PTH, and 1,25-dihydroxyvitamin D in dogs with cancer-associated hypercalcemia. Endocrinology 131(3):1157–1164

Sabatini M, Boyce B, Aufedmorte T, Bonewald L, Mundy GR (1988) Infusions of recombinant human interleukin 1α and 1β cause hypercalcemia in normal mice. Proc Natl Acad Sci USA 85:5235–5239

Sabatini M, Yates AJ, Garrett IR, Chavez J, Dunn JF, Bonewald L, Mundy GR (1990) Increased production of tumor necrosis factor by normal immune cells in a model of the humoral hypercalcemia of malignancy. Lab Invest 63(5):676–682

Saito K, Kuratomi Y, Yamamoto K, Saito T, Kuzuya T, Yoshida S, Moriyama SI, Takahashi (1981) Primary squamous cell carcinoma of the thyroid associated with marked leukocytosis and hypercalcemia. Cancer 1981 48(9):2080–2083

Salomon JC, Lynch N, Prin J (1980) Tumor transplantation in nude rats and mice. In: Sparrow S (ed) Immunodeficient animals for cancer research. Oxford University Press, New York

Sartori L, Insogna KL, Barrett PQ (1988) Renal phosphate transport in humoral hypercalcemia of malignancy. Am J Physiol 255(6/2):F1078–1084

Sato K, Fujii Y, Kasono K, Tsushima T, Shizume K (1988) Production of interleukin-1α and a parathyroid hormone-like factor by a squamous cell carcinoma of the esophagus (EC-GI) derived from a patient with hypercalcemia. J Clin Endocrinol Metab 67:592–601

Sato K, Fujii Y, Kakiuchi T, Kasono K, Imamura H, Kondo Y, Mano H, Okabe T, Asano S, Takaku F et al. (1989a) Paraneoplastic syndrome of hypercalcemia and leukocytosis caused by squamous carcinoma cells (T3M-1) producing parathyroid hormone-related protein, interleukin 1 alpha, and granulocyte colony-stimulating factor. Cancer Res 49:4740–4746

Sato K, Fujii Y, Kasono K, Ozawa M, Imamura H, Kanaji Y, Kurosawa H, Tsushima T, Shizume K (1989b) Parathyroid hormone-related protein and interleukin-1 alpha synergistically stimulate bone resorption in vitro and increase the serum calcium concentration in mice in vivo. Endocrinology 124(5):2172–2178

Sato K, Satoh T, Shizume K, Yamakawa Y, Ono Y, Demura H, Akatsu T, Takahashi N, Suda (1992) Prolonged decrease of serum calcium calcium concentration by murine gamma-interferon in hypercalcemic, human tumor (EC-GI)-bearing nude mice. Cancer Res 52(2):444–449

Sato K, Yamakawa Y, Shizume K, Satoh T, Nohtomi K, Demura H, Akatsu T, Nagata N, Kasahara T, Ohkawa H, Ohsumi K (1993) Passive immunization with anti-parathyroid hormone-related protein monoclonal antibody markedly prolongs survival time of hypercalcemic nude mice bearing transplanted human PTHrP-producing tumor. J Bone Miner Res 8(7):849–860

Saxe AW, Santora A, Norton J, Triche T, Brennan MF, Spiegel A (1985) Morphologic and functional studies of a rat hypercalcemia-associated testicular tumor maintained in cell culture. Surgery 98(6):1013–1023

Schäfer A, Raue F, Minne H, Ziegler R (1976) Dynamics of osteoclasia in rats with Walker tumor. Calcif Tissue Res [Suppl]22:368–370

Scharla SH, Minne HW, Oswald C, Lempert UG, Schmidt-Gayk H, Ziegler R (1989) The hypercalcemic Walker carcinosarcoma 256 of the rat causes an increase in serum 1,25-dihydroxyvitamin D_3. Bone Miner 6:155–164

Scharla SH, Minne HW, Lempert UG, Krieg P, Rappel S, Maurer E, Grohe U, Ziegler R (1991) Osteolytic activity of Walker carcinosarcoma 256 is due to parathyroid hormone-related protein (PTHrP). Horm Metab Res 23(2):66–69

Schilling T, Blind E, Wagner H, Raue F, Ziegler R (1993a) Dexamethasone decreases parathyroid hormone-related protein secretion in-vitro but not in-vivo in the rat Walker carcinosarcoma 256. Calcif Tissue Int 5[Suppl 1]:S71

Schilling T, Blind E, Raue F, Ziegler R (1993b) Determination of the plasma half-life of parathyroid hormone-related protein using the rat Walker carcinosarcoma 256. Eur J Clin Invest 23[Suppl 1]:A10

Schilling T, Pecherstorfer M, Blind E, Leidig G, Ziegler R, Raue F (1993c) Parathyroid hormone-related protein (PTHrP) does not regulate 1,25-dihydroxyvitamin D serum levels in hypercalcemia of malignancy. J Clin Endocrinol Metab 76: 801–803
Schmidt-Gayk H, Löhrke H, Fischkal A, Goertller K, Hofmann F (1979) Urinary cyclic AMP and bone histology in Walker carcinosarcoma: evidence of parathyroid hormone-like activity. Eur J Cancer 15:1211–1218
Schmidt-Gayk H, Lohrke H, Hesse B, Fischkal A, Goerttler K (1983) Electrolyte and glucose metabolism in VX-2 carcinoma of the rabbit. Eur J Cancer Clin Oncol 19(7):951–957
Seyberth HW, Hubbard WC, Oelz O, Sweetman BJ, Watson JT, Oates JA (1977) Prostaglandin-mediated hypercalcemia in the VX2 carcinoma-bearing rabbit. Prostaglandins 14:319–331
Shevrin DH, Lad TE, Kukreja SC (1987) Effect of epidermal growth factor infusion on serum and urine calcium in mice. J Bone Miner Res 2(4):297–301
Shipley PJ, Shevrin DH, Kukreja SC (1988) Increased renal calcium reabsorption in an animal model of hypercalcemia of human malignancy. J Bone Miner Res 3(5):555–560
Simpkins H, Lehman JM, Mazurkiewicz JE, Davis BH (1991) A morphological nad phenotypic analysis of Walker 256 cells. Cancer Res 51:1334–1338
Sowers JR, Barrett JD (1982) Hormonal changes associated with hypertension in neoplasia-induced hypercalcemia. Am J Physiol 242(5):E330–334
Spiegel AM, Saxe AW, Deftos LJ, Brennan MF (1983) Humoral hypercalcemia caused by a rat Leydig-cell tumor is associated with suppressed parathyroid hormone secretion and increased urinary cAMP excretion. Horm Metab Res 15(6):299–304
Steele TD, Bryant HU, Malven PV, Yim GKW (1988) Nocturnal depletion of hypothalamic dynorphin in anorexic Walker-256 tumor-bearing rats. Pharmacol Biochem Behav 29:541–545
Stern PH, Krieger NS, Nissenson RA, Williams RD, Winkler ME, Derynck R, Strewler GJ (1985) Human transforming growth factor-alpha stimulates bone resorption in vitro. J Clin Invest 76(5):2016–2019
Stewart HL, Snell KC, Dunham LJ, Schlyen SM (1959) In: Atlas of tumor pathology, section XII, fasc 40, Air Force Institute of Pathology, Washington DC, pp 216–271
Stewart AF, Horst R, Deftos LJ, Cadman EC, Lang R, Broadus AE (1980) Biochemical evaluation of patients with cancer-associated hypercalcemia; evidence for humoral and nonhumoral groups. N Engl J Med 303:1377–1383
Stoica G, Koestner A, Capen CC (1983) Characterization of *N*-ethyl-*N*-nitrosourea-induced mammary tumors in the rat. Am J Pathol 110(2):161–169
Strewler GJ, Nissenson RA (1990) Peptide mediators of hypercalcemia in malignancy. Annu Rev Med 41:35–44
Strewler GJ, Williams RD, Nissenson RA (1983) Human renal carcinoma cells produce hypercalcemia in the nude mouse and a novel protein recognized by parathyroid hormone receptors. J Clin Invest 71(3):769–774
Strewler GJ, Wronski TJ, Halloran BP, Miller SC, Leung SC, Williams RD, Nissenson RA (1986) Pathogenesis of hypercalcemia in nude mice bearing a human renal carcinoma. Endocrinology 119(1):303–310
Suzuki K, Yamada S (1991) Ascites sarcoma 180, an animal model of humoral hypercalcemia of malignancy, produces a factor(s) exhibiting potent bone-resorbing activity without any parathyroid hormone-like activity. Bone Miner 14(1):1–13
Takeuchi T, Takeuchi H, Hoshino R, Ohmi K (1982) Rhabdomyosarcoma-induced hypercalcemia in a nude mouse. Cancer 50(1):94–96

Tam CS, Heersche JN, Santora A, Spiegel AM (1984) Skeletal response in rats following the implantation of hypercalcemia-producing Leydig cell tumors. Metabolism 33(1):50–53

Tashjian AH, Voelkel EF, Levine L, Goldhaber P (1972) Evidence that the bone resorption-stimulating factor produced by mouse fibrosarcoma cells is prostaglandin E_2: a new model for the hypercalcemia of cancer. J Exp Med 136:1329

Tashjian AH, Voelkel EF, Goldhaber P, Levine L (1973) Successful treatment of hypercalcemia by indomethacin in mice bearing a prostalgandin producing fibrosarcoma. Prostaglandins 3:515–524

Tashjian AH, Voelkel EF, Goldhaber P, Levine L (1974) Prostaglandins, calcium metabolism and cancer. Fed Proc 33:81–87

Tashjian AH, Voelkel EF, Levine L (1977a) Plasma concentrations of 13,14-dihydro-15-keto-prostaglandin E2 in rabbits bearing the VX2 carcinoma: effects of hydrocortisone and indomethacin. Prostaglandins 14:309–317

Tashjian AH, Voelkel EF, Goldhaber P, Levine L (1977b) Effects of hydrocortisone on the hypercalcemia and plasma levels of 13,14-dihydro-15-keto prostaglandin E_2 in mice bearing the $HSDM_1$ fibrosarcoma. Biochem Biophys Res Commun 74: 199–207

Tashjian A, Voelkel E, Robinson D, Levine L (1984) Dietary menhaden oil lowers plasma prostaglandins and calcium in mice bearing the prostalgandin-producing $HSDM_1$ fibrosarcoma. J Clin Invest 74:2042–2048

Taylor JM, Simpson RU (1992) Inhibition of cancer cell growth by calcium channel antagonists in the athymic mouse. Cancer Res 52(9):2413–2418

Thompson DD, Seedor JG, Fisher JE, Rosenblatt M, Rodan GA (1988) Direct action of the parathyroid hormone-like human hypercalcemic factor on bone. Proc Natl Acad Sci USA 85(15):5673–5677

Torres R, Diaz Diego EM, de la Piedra C, Rapado A (1992) Plasma of Walker-256 carcinosarcoma bearing rats contains parathormone related peptide. Horm Metab Res 24:246–247

Torring O, Turner RT, Carter WB, Firek AF, Jacobs CA, Health H III (1992) Inhibition by human interleukin-1 alpha of parathyroid hormone-related peptide effects on renal calcium and phosphorus metabolism in the rat. Endocrinology 131(1):5–13

Troyer H, Sowers JR, Babich E (1982) Leydig cell tumor induced hypercalcemia in the Fischer rat: morphometric and histochemical evidence for a humoral factor that activates osteoclasts. Am J Pathol 108(3):284–290

Voelkel EF, Tashjian AH Jr, Franklin R, Wasserman E, Levine L (1975) Hypercalcemia and tumor-prostaglandins: the VX2 carcinoma model in the rabbit. Metabolism 24(8):973–986

Wagner H, Blind E, Raue F (1993) Secretion and storage of parathyroid hormone-related protein is decreased by vitamin D and glucocorticoids in a C-cell line and in the rat Walker carcinosarcoma 256. Exp Clin Endocrinol 101[Suppl 1]:174

Warrell RP Jr, Bockman RS, Coonley CJ, Isaacs M, Staszewski H (1984) Gallium nitrate inhibits calcium resorption from bone and is effective treatment for cancer-related hypercalcemia. J Clin Invest 73:1487–1490

Watanabe K, Tanaka Y, Morimoto I, Yahata K, Zeki K, Fumihira T, Yamashita U, Eto S (1990) Interleukin-4 as a potent inhibitor of bone resorption. Biochem Biophys Res Commun 172:1035–1041

Weir EC, Burtis WJ, Morris CA, Brady TG, Insogna KL (1988a) Isolation of 16000-dalton parathyroid hormone-like proteins from two animal tumors causing humoral hypercalcemia of malignancy. Endocrinology 123(6):2744–2751

Weir EC, Insogna KL, Brownstein DG, Bander NH, Broadus AE (1988b) In vitro adenylate cyclase-stimulating activity predicts the occurrence of humoral hypercalcemia of malignancy in nude mice. J Clin Invest 81(3):818–821

Weir EC, Norrdin RW, Matus RE, Brooks MB, Broadus AE, Mitnick M, Johnston SD, Insogna KL (1988c) Humoral hypercalcemia of malignancy in canine lymphosarcoma. Endocrinology 122(2):602–608
Weiss J, Walker ST, Fallon M, Goldfarb S (1986) In vivo and in vitro effects of WR-2721 in experimental hypercalcemia in the rat. J Pharmacol Exp Ther 238(3):969–973
Weller RE, Melcon D (1978) Malignant hypercalcemia in a dog with lymphosarcoma. Mod Vet Pract 59:901–903
Wilson JR, Merrick H, Woodward ER (1961) Hypercalcemia simulating hyperparathyroidism induced by VX-2 carcinoma in rabbits. Ann Surg 154:485
Wilson JR, Merrick H, Vogel SD, Woodward ER (1965) Hyperparathyroid-like state in rabbits with the VX-2 carcinoma: further studies. Am Surg 31:145
Winchell HS, Sanchez PD, Watanabe CK et al. (1970) Visualization of tumors in humans using ^{67}Ga-citrate and the anger whole-body scanner, scintillation camera and tomographic scanner. J Nucl Med 11:459–466
Wingen F, Eichmann T, Manegold C, Krempien B (1986) Effects of bisphosphonic acids on tumor-induced bone destruction in the rat. J Cancer Res Clin Oncol 111:35–41
Wolfe H, Bitman W, Voelkel E, Griffiths HJ, Tashjian AH (1978) Systemic effects of the VX2 carcinoma on the osseous skeleton. Lab Invest 38:208–215
Yamamoto I, Kitamura N, Aoki J, Kawamura J, Dokoh S (1987) Circulating 1,25-dihydroxyvitamin D concentrations in patients with renal cell carcinoma-associated hypercalcemia are rarely suppressed. J Clin Endocrinol Metab 64:175–179
Yates AJ, Gutierrez GE, Smolens P, Travis PS, Katz MS, Aufdemorte TB, Boyce BF, Hymer TK, Poser JW, Mundy GR (1988) Effects of a synthetic peptide of a parathyroid hormone-related protein on calcium homeostasis, renal tubular calcium reabsorption, and bone metabolism in vivo and in vitro in rodents. J Clin Invest 81(3):932–938
Yates AJ, Boyce BF, Favarato G, Aufdemorte TB, Marcelli C, Kester MB, Walker R, Langton BC, Bonewald LF, Mundy GR (1992) Expression of human transforming growth factor alpha by Chinese hamster ovarian tumors in nude mice causes hypercalcemia and increased osteoclastic bone resorption. J Bone Miner Res 7(7):847–853
Yoneda T, Alsina MA, Chavez JB, Bonewald L, Nishimura R, Mundy GR (1991) Evidence that tumor necrosis factor plays a pathogenetic role in the paraneoplastic syndromes of cachexia, hypercalcemia, and leukocytosis in a human tumor in nude mice. J Clin Invest 87(3):977–985
Yoneda T, Nakai M, Moriyama K, Scott L, Ida N, Kunitomo T, Mundy GR (1993) Neutralizing antibodies to human interleukin 6 reverse hypercalcemia associated with a human squamous cacinoma. Cancer Res 53(4):737–740
Young DM, Fioravanti JL, Prieur DJ, Ward JM (1976) Hypercalcemic VX-2 carcinoma in rabbits: a clinicopathologic study. Lab Invest 35(1):30–46
Young DM, Ward JM, Prieur DJ (1978) Hypercalcemia of malignancy. Animal model: VX-2 carcinoma of rabbits. Am J Pathol 93(2):619–622
Yuhas JM, Storer JB (1969) Differential chemoprotection of normal and malignant tissues. J Natl Cancer Inst 42:331–335
Yuhas JM, Spellman JM, Culo F (1980) The role of WR-2721 in radiotherapy and/or chemotherapy. Cancer Clin Trials 3:211–216

Morphological Characteristics of Tumors with Humoral Hypercalcemia of Malignancy: Functional Morphology of PTHrP

A. Turzynski[1], S. Baumgart[2], B. Bauch[2], and M. Dietel[1]

[1] Institute of Pathology, University Hospital Charité, Humboldt University, Schumannstraße 20/21, 10117 Berlin, Germany
[2]Institute of General Pathology and Anatomy, Christian Albrechts University Kiel, Michaelisstraße 11, 24105 Kiel, Germany

Introduction

The appearance of defined paraneoplastic syndromes in the context of tumor illnesses is a well-known phenomenon. Paraneoplastic syndrome is the term used to indicate those systematic clinically observable effects brought on by malignant growths that are not locally determined. They are dependent on the presence of the tumor, and can at least temporarily disappear after excision of the tumor. They show up in the form of neurological, hematological or endocrine disturbances, and can manifest themselves as dermal, muscle, joint or bone alterations. Thus, from the point of view of etiology, a whole series of illnesses are subsumed under this concept. The activation of a latent viral infection by leukemia or malignant lymphomas, for instance, can lead to progressive multifocal leukoencephalopathy. Autoimmune processes are responsible for the occurrence of myasthenia gravis in the course of thymoma, or of Lambert-Eaton syndrome with bronchial carcinoma. The clinically most remarkable are the endocrine paraneoplastic syndromes. These are brought about by the excessive production of proteo-, peptide or steroid hormones. The hormone production caused by the tumor or its metastases leads only then to observable symptoms, when the type and amount of the hormone overwhelms the body's intrinsic counterregulation mechanisms. However, strictly speaking, the concept of endocrine paraneoplastic syndrome, or sometimes paraendocrine syndrome, is reserved for those tumor manifestations in which the original tissue from which the tumor derives lacks the ability to produce the particular hormone. Such an ectopic hormone production therefore represents a newly acquired characteristic of the tumor.

The most important endocrine paraneoplastic syndrome is the humoral hypercalcemia of malignancy (HHM). Its claim to importance is not only based on the fact that it is clinically the most frequent paraneoplastic syndrome, but also because it represents a serious complication of a tumor disease. The syndrome often resists therapeutic measures, and is thus not uncommonly fatal. The possible hormonal factors that come into question as the cause of the disturbance of the calcium homeostasis are many, and reflect the diversity of calciotropic effectors. They include parathyroid hormone (PTH), PTH-like proteins, vitamin D_3, cytokines, and growth factors. Within tumor-associated hypercalcemia syndromes, the hypercalcemia brought on by ossary metastasis is differentiated, in which the calcium mobilization due to local bone resorption leads to a rise in serum calcium levels. As opposed to HHM, this form of hypercalcemia represents a local tumor complication, in which, however, paracrine factors often play a role.

Of the factors that induce HHM, parathyroid hormone related protein (PTHrP) is the most frequent. This hormone was first identified, and its structure clarified, in squamous cell, breast, and renal cell carcinomas in 1987, and in the first 13 amino acids of the N-terminus shows a 60% sequence homology with parathormone (Moseley et al. 1987). This limited homology nonetheless allows PTHrP to integrate with the PTH/PTHrP receptor, and its high affinity thus results in disruptions of the calcium homeostasis.

The following overview of the morphological findings on tumors with HHM is restricted to the role of PTHrP and is based on the literature and on results we have garnered. It follows from the definition of endocrine paraneoplastic syndrome that it is essential also to consider the original tissue of the tumor for an expression of this proteohormone.

Methodological Aspects

The correlation of morphological observations in situ with functional findings in vitro or in vivo is the task of functional morphology. In histological sections a gene product can be visualized at two levels:

- At the mRNA level, which can be demonstrated by in situ hybridization (ISH)
- At the protein level, which can be demonstrated by immunohistochemical procedures

The broad applicability of immunohistochemistry and in situ hybridization is based both on the specificity of the antibodies or gene probes used, and on the sensitivity of the detection methods. However, there are both biological and technical limitations to these methods. In the field of endocrinology, primarily for biological reasons, the use of either method to demonstrate a gene product must be complemented by application of the other method. It is a mistake, therefore, to see the two methods as alternatives. The pool of intracellular hormones results from labile steady-state conditions that reflect the simultaneous processes of de novo synthesis, storage, intracellular degradation and secretion. Exclusive application of immunohistochemical methods might give results seemingly in contradiction to functional findings (Dietel and Dorn-Quint 1980), contradictions that could only be resolved by application of mRNA detection. Under maximal stimulation in endocrine active cells there could well be no hormone visible, since the post-Golgi pool has been completely released. On the other hand, in situ hybridization of mRNA would give a strong signal, since in this case it would reflect the elevated hormone synthesis.

Furthermore, since immunohistochemistry alone gives no information as to the source of the hormone, it provides no way of ruling out the possibility that the immunoreactivity observed may be due to hormone uptake into the cell, as opposed to the production of the hormone within the cell. In situ hybridization, though, can answer this question.

Another important point is that a gene product might be manifested in several molecular forms. Indeed, PTHrP has been shown to exhibit a molecular diversity due both to alternative mRNA splicing (Mangin et al. 1988; Suva et al. 1989; Thiede et al. 1988) and to posttranscriptional processing, e.g., glycosylation (Wu et al. 1991). Antibodies might recognize only a subset of the possible molecular forms, thus leading to false-negative results. This is especially true for monoclonal antibodies.

Lastly, the positive demonstration of a sequence-specific RNA for a possible secretion product must not be considered conclusive evidence for its actual synthesis and/or release. Recently, truncated gene transcripts of the vasopressin and opiomelanocortin gene were demonstrated in testis that, being nonfunctional, could not in fact have synthesized the hormone (Ivell 1993).

Unfortunately, the technical limitations of these morphological methods often prevent their simultaneous application on one tissue sample. Hormone production is therefore only seldom demonstrable at both levels. As a rule, material most easily available, such as archival samples in pathology departments, is only processed for routine paraffin histology. Because of the high instability of messenger RNA, it is rarely possible to use this material for in situ hybridization studies. Only high copy gene transcripts present in cells such as insulin, and glucagon mRNA in pancreatic islet (Shorrock et al. 1991), or calcitonin mRNA in medullary thyroid carcinoma (le Guellec et al. 1993), can be detected in paraffin-embedded material. Nevertheless, it should be remembered that the demonstrated mRNA represents only a part of the gene transcripts present in the cell at the time of the removal of the tissue. Since the speed of tissue fixation and thereby of the RNase inactivation varies with different tissue types, the success of mRNA in situ hybridization depends primarily on the inhibition of RNA degradation. The introduction of single-stranded oligonucleotides and riboprobes greatly improved the sensitivity of the detection procedure. Nonetheless, the staining obtained may still vary extensively depending on the method of tissue processing. Koji and Brenner (1993) showed differences in the detectability of estrogen receptor (ER) mRNA in the rhesus monkey uterus, differences that depended largely upon the fixation protocol: while ER-specific mRNA is strongly demonstrable in the laminae functionalis of samples that are freshly frozen, cryosectioned, and then fixed in formaldehyde or actone, and basalis and the myometrium are demonstrable to the same extent, the mRNA staining obtained is limited to the functionalis and is only weakly present in the basalis when the tissue block is fixed prior to the cryosectioning. In myometrium, even after two-step formaldehyde fixation, no ER mRNA was demonstrable. This underlines the fact that relevant in situ hybridization results can only be expected after appropriate and optimal tissue processing.

For these reasons there has been only one study on the in situ detection of PTHrP mRNA in tumors (Heath et al. 1990). In most ISH studies, animal, experimental, normal, and fetal tissues are investigated. Thus, the localization of PTHrP in tumors is predominantly based on immunohistochemistry.

For the immunohistochemical detection of PTH and PTHrP, several antibodies raised against different epitopes are available. Since PTH and PTHrP have some homologous sequences in their N-terminus, it is possible that antibodies directed against this portion might cross-react with both peptides. Indeed, when the first radioimmunoassay for PTH (Berson and Yalow 1966) was established, supposedly elevated PTH was detected in sera of patients with humoral hypercalcemia of malignancy caused by lung carcinomas. In early immunohistochemical studies the existence of PTH immunoreactivity or a PTH-like substance was described, and this supported the hypothesis that HHM is due to ectopic PTH production (see Martin et al. 1989, for review).

After the PTHrP had been isolated, cloned, and sequenced, specific non-cross-reacting antisera could be raised. Consequently, these antisera differentiate between PTH and PTHrP. Although there are recent observations of PTH production by a small cell lung carcinoma (Yoshimoto et al. 1989) and a carcinoma of the ovary (Nussbaum et al. 1990) the ectopic paraneoplastic production of PTH by malignomas must be considered a rare event. PTHrP remains recognized as the most frequent causative factor of HHM.

In subsequent morphological studies, PTHrP was shown to be produced in tumors far more frequently than expected, considering the relatively rare incidence of HHM. PTHrP production was noted particularly in tumor types known to be associated with HHM, such as squamous carcinomas or breast carcinomas. Unlike other paracrine syndromes (e.g., Cushing's syndrome brought on by ectopic ACTH production, or Bartter-Schwarz syndrome caused by inappropriate vasopressin secretion; both associated mostly with small cell lung carcinomas), expression of PTHrP is common to a variety of tumors with various histogeneses and differentiations.

Since even malignant tumors exhibit features of their tissue of origin or regain features of earlier developmental states, it became necessary to specify the locations of physiological PTHrP production. In particular, the ability to localize PTHrP by morphological detection methods led to a more comprehensive understanding of PTHrP and its possible functions in physiological and pathological conditions.

PTHrP in Tumor, Normal, and Fetal Tissues of Various Organs

Skin, Skin Appendages, and Related Tumors

PTHrP production is most frequently found in squamous cell carcinomas. Indeed, PTHrP was purified for the first time from the BEN cell line (Moseley et al. 1987; Martin et al. 1989), which was established from a squamous lung carcinoma (Ellison et al. 1975). Previously, a protein acting similar to PTH had been noted in cultured normal human keratinocytes (Merendino et al. 1986). Subsequently, PTHrP immunoreactivity was described in keratinocytes of keratinizing and nonkeratinizing squamous epithelia by several groups (Hayman et al. 1989; Danks et al. 1989; Atillasoy et al. 1991; Kitazawa et al. 1991; S. Kitazawa et al. 1992). Expression of this protein is especially prominent throughout the spinous layer of keratinizing epithelia, whereas basal and parabasal cells show less or no staining (Fig. 1). Using a polyclonal rabbit antiserum raised against the N-terminal peptide, staining of the granular layer was variable and no staining was seen in the surface keratin (Hayman et al. 1989). Among the skin appendages, strong immunoreactivity is present in the inner sheath of hair follicles, but not in the associated sebaceous glands or in sweat glands (Hayman et al. 1989; Kitazawa et al. 1991). In addition, nonkeratinizing epithelia in the esophagus, tongue, vagina and cervix uteri show strong immunoreactivity.

Presumably, the production of PTHrP in the normal skin by far exceeds the production of PTH in the parathyroids (Rosol and Capen 1992), even though, under physiological conditions, at best only a small amount of PTHrP appears in the systemic circulation. Thus, it has been suggested that PTHrP may play a local role as an auto- or paracrine-acting growth and/or differentiation factor. The immunohistochemical pattern of PTHrP immunoreactivity indicates a close relationship both with the processes that transform basal progenitor cells into squamous epithelia and with the maturation of keratinocytes. This functional morphological interpretation is supported by the recent demonstration (Orloff et al. 1992) of:

1. PTHrP secretion by cultured nonmalignant keratinocytes in a regulated manner
2. PTH/PTHrP-binding sites on keratinocytes
3. Intracellular postreceptor signal transduction events, namely a rapid transient and dose-dependent increase in intracellular Ca^{2+} concentration

Although the precise function of PTHrP in skin remains to be established, it has been shown to inhibit proliferation and induce differentiation in human cultured neonatal keratinocytes (Holick et al. 1988).

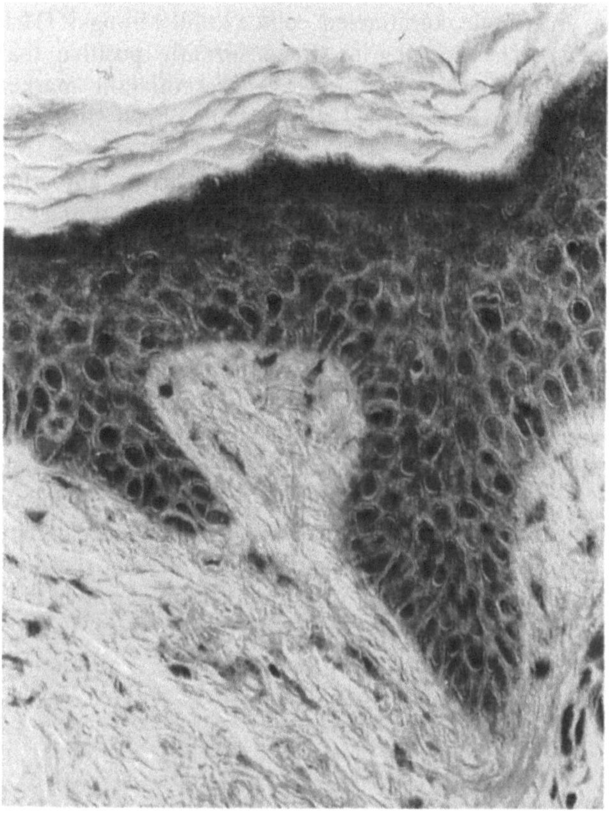

Fig. 1. Localization of PTHrP in normal skin. PTHrP immunoreactivity in the keratinocytes gradually increases with keratinization. Polyclonal anti-PTHrP (34–53), avidin-biotin complex technique, nuclear counterstain with hematoxylin, differential interference contrast optics, ×400

In pathologically altered tissues, PTHrP can be found in lesions exhibiting a squamous or hair follicle differentiation, which is in agreement with the findings mentioned above. The expression is not restricted to lesions of epidermal origin, but is also seen in squamous metaplasia of bronchial and transitional epithelia (Kitazawa et al. 1991), and even in skin and hair follice elements of a cystic teratoma of the testis (Hayman et al. 1989).

Given these findings, it is not in itself remarkable that PTHrP expression was detected in squamous carcinomas of variable localization. Squamous carcinomas of the skin (Hayman et al. 1989), of the oral or pharyngeal mucous epithelium, of the esophagus (Tachimori et al. 1991), of the female genital tract (S. Kitazawa et al. 1992), and particularly of the lower respiratory tract (Heath et al. 1990; Ralston et al. 1991; Kitazawa et al. 1991) frequently produce PTHrP.

By immunohistochemistry squamous carcinomas also show a staining pattern that varies depending on the differentiation: particularly cells in areas of keratinization and single keratinized cells exhibit strong PTHrP immunopositivity (Fig. 2). The staining is so consistently positive that the use of PTHrP expression as a histological differentiation marker for squamous differentiation in pathological diagnosis has been suggested (Hayman et al. 1989).

There is increasing evidence that PTHrP might serve as an autocrine growth factor also in tumors. The proliferation of the PTHrP-secreting cell line BEN-57 is significantly inhibited when autocrine effects of PTHrP are specifically blocked by antibodies either against N-terminal or midregional PTHrP or by a surplus of the PTHrP antagonist PTHrP(7–34) (Burton and Knight 1992). Transforming growth factor alpha was shown to stimulate PTHrP secretion, and may be involved in an autocrine regulation loop for malignant keratinocyte proliferation.

As of yet, no obvious correlation between the histological pattern or intensity of PTHrP staining and the patient's serum calcium levels has been established. However, R. Kitazawa et al. (1992) report that in squamous carcinomas of the uterine cervix the strength of PTHrP immunoreactivity correlates to a certain extent with the development of the stromal reaction. The intensity of PTHrP staining was strong in tumors of the scirrhous type

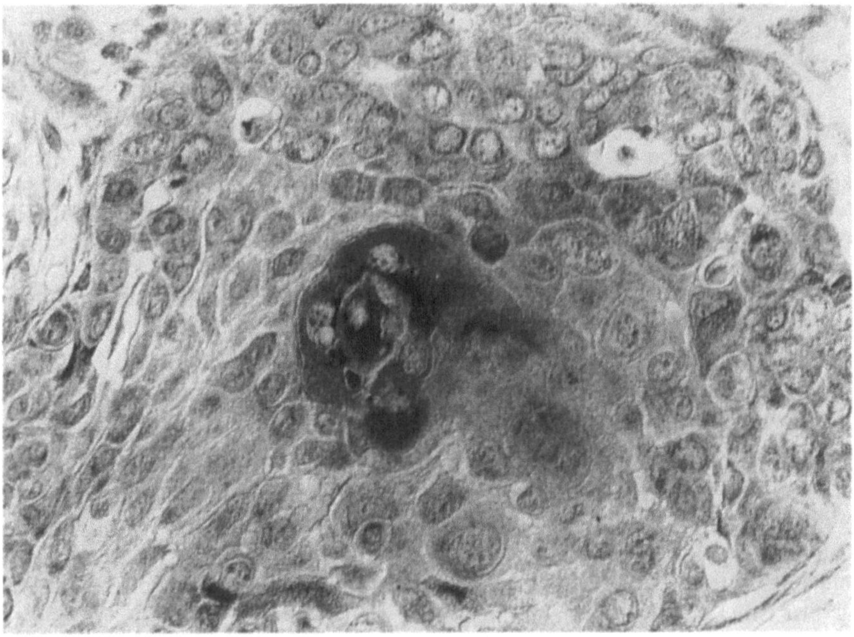

Fig. 2. Localization of PTHrP in a squamous cell carcinoma. Intense immunoreactivity is prominent in areas of keratinization. Polyclonal anti-PTHrP (34–53), avidin-biotin complex technique, nuclear counterstain with hematoxylin, differential interference contrast optics, ×400

whereas tumors of the medullary type tended to show a weaker staining. Consequently, the two invasive carcinomas associated with HHM that were included in this study exhibited a strong stromal reaction, while the majoriy of carcinomas without HHM showed a medullary growth pattern. These morphological findings are supported by in vitro investigations, in which the interaction between fibroblasts and squamous carcinoma cells was investigated with reference to PTHrP secretion (Hoekman et al. 1990). Different squamous carcinoma cell lines were shown to markedly increase their PTHrP production and secretion when they were cocultured with fibroblasts. It is clear that this effect is mediated by a soluble factor of the fibroblasts, since a direct cell-to-cell contact between carcinoma cells and fibroblasts is not necessary to bring about the effect. Fibroblast-conditioned medium alone, on the other hand, failed to elicit this effect. It is likely that the fibroblastic PTHrP-inducing factor is liberated as a response to a factor of the carcinoma cells that is likewise soluble. There is a delay of 2–3 days after coculturing before the onset of elevated PTHrP secretion occurs. It is interesting to note that cultured normal dermal fibroblasts also express functional PTH/PTHrP receptors (Gupta et al. 1991). This complex epithelial-mesenchymal interaction may be involved in the development of HHM. The hypothesis might then be put forward that HHM results not only from disturbances in tumor cell function, but may be caused by close intercellular (stromal-epithelial) interactions that gain particular importance in invasive squamous cell – and perhaps other – carcinomas.

Mammary Gland and Breast Cancer

PTHrP can also be demonstrated in the breast under both physiological and pathological conditions. By means of radioimmunoassays, the highest concentrations of PTHrP in physiological body fluids has been found in milk. The levels are approximately 1000 times higher than the serum concentrations measured in patients with HHM (Bundayr et al. 1989; Bucht et al. 1992; Yamamoto et al. 1992). It has been convincingly demonstrated that the epithelia of a non-lactating breast expresses no PTHrP. Only in lactating breast is PTHrP expression found. One hormonal agent that causes PTHrP induction is prolactin (Thiede 1989). The functional significance of PTHrP is to a large extent unknown, although it appears to contribute to the calcium mobilization in milk (Barlet et al. 1992). In primary epithelial cultures culled from lactating breasts, the secretion of biologically active PTHrP could be demonstrated (Ferrari et al. 1992). It was determined in this context that the PTHrP secretion by breast epithelia was in inverse proportion to the proliferation rate.

Of all the malignancies,.mammary carcinomas have the highest incidence of tumor-associated hypercalcemia. On the one hand, this is due to the high rate of bone metastases in mammary carcinomas. On the other hand, a high percentage of PTHrP expression in mammary carcinomas of various histological types can be identified. While Danks et al. (1989) found PTHrP in one of six mammary carcinomas, in 61 cases in an immunohistological study of 102 invasive mammary carcinomas PTHrP 1–34 immunoreactivity was demonstrated with the help of rabbit antiserum (Southby et al. 1990). Similarly, Bundred et al. (1992) found PTHrP immunopositivity after application of a rabbit anti-PTHrP 37–67 antiserum in approximately 60% of 155 cases of early breast cancer. Based on our own observations, the percentage of PTHrP-positive tumors could well be even higher. With the help of a polyclonal, affinity-purified anti-PTHrP(34–58) antibody (Oncogen/Dianova), administered in concentrations of 1 μg/ml, more than 90% of the approximately 100 unselected mammary carcinomas investigated showed PTHrP formation (paper in preparation).

Immunoreactivity is confined to the cytoplasm of tumor cells usually exhibiting a granular staining pattern (Fig. 3). In these cells and tumor areas with very strong immunopositivity, the staining appears to be diffusely cytoplasmatic, and only the nucleus is left unstained. This might be due to the limited spatial resolution of light microscopy. In most cases other tumor cells in the same section showing less staining support the hypothesis that PTHrP is generally stored in vesicles. This can be considered the morphological prerequisite for the secretion of PTHrP by the tumor cells.

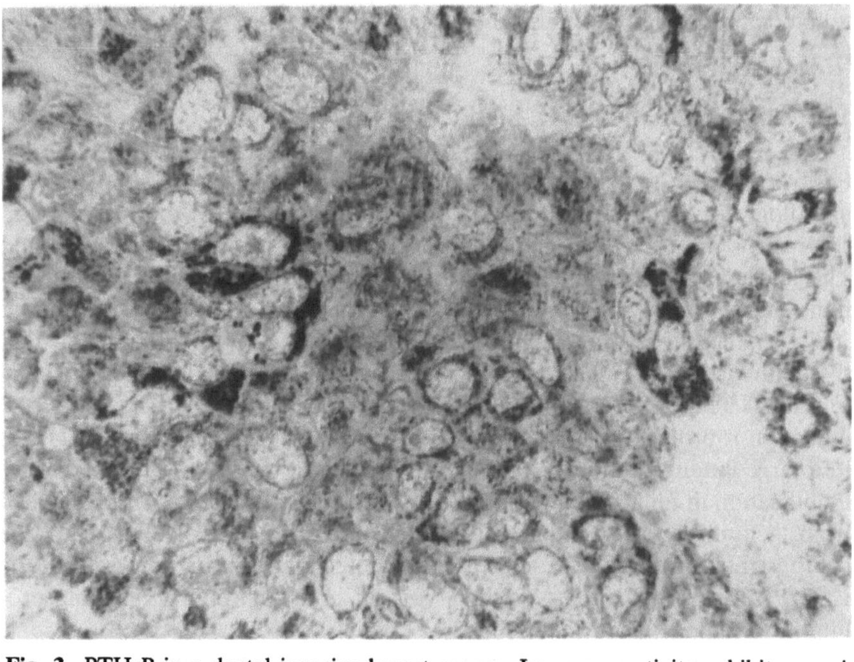

Fig. 3. PTHrP in a ductal invasive breast cancer. Immunoreactivity exhibits a vesicular pattern. Polyclonal anti-PTHrP (34–53), avidin-biotin complex technique, nuclear counterstain with hematoxylin, ×1000

The distribution of PTHrP-positive cells ranges from a few cells, mostly confined to the margins of a solid tumor area, to staining of every tumor cell in a section. In general, the invasive portions show a markedly higher staining for PTHrP than the intraductal portions (Fig. 4). This was stated first by Southby et al. (1990). It seems possible that PTHrP contributes to the invasive ability of a tumor, although this hypothesis has yet to bet supported by experimental results.

Given the large percentage of PTHrP-producing tumors among all breast cancers – whether 60% or 90% – no prediction based on immunohistochemistry can be made concerning the development of HHM. Attempts to correlate PTHrP staining with known prognostic factors (e.g., age, tumor size, histological type and grade, nodal status, estrogen and progesterone status in breast cancer) have so far failed to show statistical significance. Nevertheless, among tumor size, stage, and lymph node status, PTHrP immunopositivity appears to be prognostic for the development of skeletal metastases. Bone metastases secondary to breast cancer were shown to express PTHrP with a much higher frequency (12/13 cases, 92%) compared with metastases in non-bone sites (3/18 cases, 17%) (Powell et al. 1991). The difference was statistically highly significant. Production of PTHrP as a bone-targeting agent may contribute to the ability of breast cancer to seed

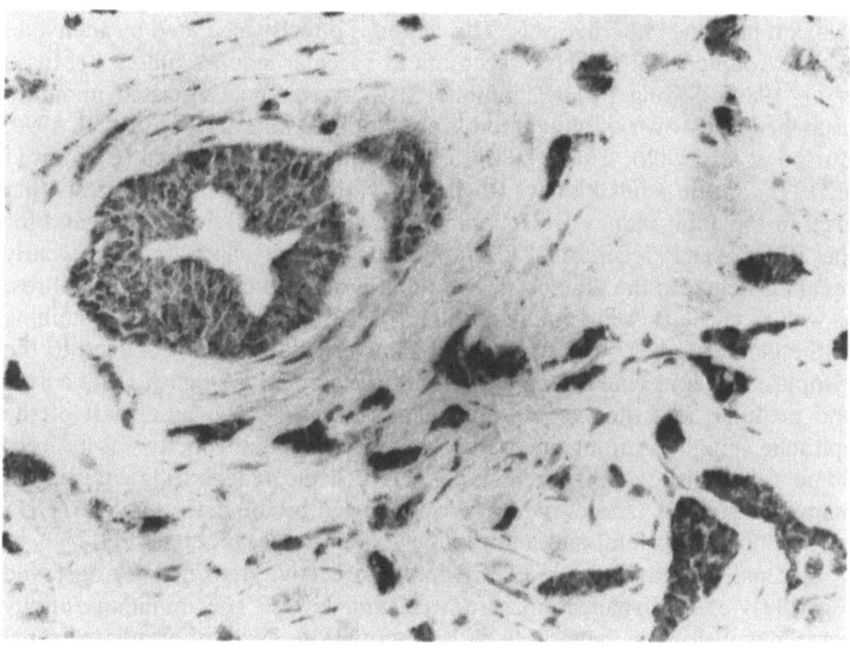

Fig. 4. PTHrP in an invasive breast cancer. Immunoreactivity is most prominent in the invasive cells. Polyclonal anti-PTHrP (34–53), avidin-biotin complex technique, nuclear counterstain with hematoxylin, ×400

bone metastases, but may also reflect the activity of PTHrP-inducing factors present in bone or bone marrow. In several studies, elevated serum PTHrP levels were demonstrated in patients with solid tumors and hypercalcemia irrespective of bone involvement (Burtis et al. 1990; Henderson et al. 1990; Kao et al. 1990; Grill et al. 1991; Blind et al. 1992). The actual causal relationship between PTHrP production and skeletal metastases remains to be established.

Kidney and Renal Cell Carcinoma

The kidneys are one of the main target organs of PTH actions. High-affinity receptors for PTH have been detected in preparations of cortical plasma membranes, and PTHrP was shown to bind to these receptors with equal affinity (Caulfield et al. 1990). The PTH/PTHrP receptor was recently cloned and sequenced from opossum kidney cells (Jüppner et al. 1991). With seven membrane-spanning regions this receptor exhibits some structural similarities to the calcitonin receptor (Lin et al. 1991) and appears to be coupled to several signal transduction pathways. PTHrP was shown to exert PTH-like effects in kidneys in vivo and in vitro as well as in cultured kidney cells (Zhou et al. 1989; Pizurki et al. 1988). For some effects even a higher potency of PTHrP was reported (Ellis et al. 1990). In addition to their effects on renal epithelial cells, both hormones act as potent vasorelaxant in kidney microvessels. This action is directly mediated by adenylate cyclase coupled PTH/PTHrP receptors in vascular smooth muscles (Musso et al. 1989). Strong PTHrP immunoreactivity was demonstrated immunohistochemically over a long period in developing kidneys (Moniz et al. 1990; Burton et al. 1990a). This is still present in the postpartal organ (Campos et al. 1991) and in adult kidneys (own observations), a fact that suggests that even in the adult kidney PTHrP might actually be a physiological ligand for the PTH/PTHrP receptor. PTHrP immunopositivity appears in the early renal blastema, in the glomeruli, and tubules of the meso- and metanephros, as well as in the calyceal epithelium. During further maturation, the staining of the glomeruli is lost. Staining exhibits a vesicular pattern confined to the cytoplasm of epithelial cell in all parts of the tubular system in renal cortex and medulla, and the vesicles are mainly located in the basal part of the epithelia (Fig. 5). Among ducts and tubules some heterogeneity was noticed. Some tubules stained strongly for PTHrP, while neighboring tubules remained unstained. These findings are supported by the detection of PTHrP-specific mRNA in fetal and adult kidneys (Selvanayagam et al. 1991).

In renal cell carcinomas PTHrP immunoreactivity is regularly observed regardless of disturbances in serum calcium levels. The immunopositivity correlates well with the degree of differentiation. Well-differentiated renal carcinomas exhibit strong immunoreactivity (Fig. 6), while undifferentiated (grade III) tumors show a much weaker staining (Fig. 7). Particularly in grade II renal cell carcinomas this trend is evident, since parts of the tumors

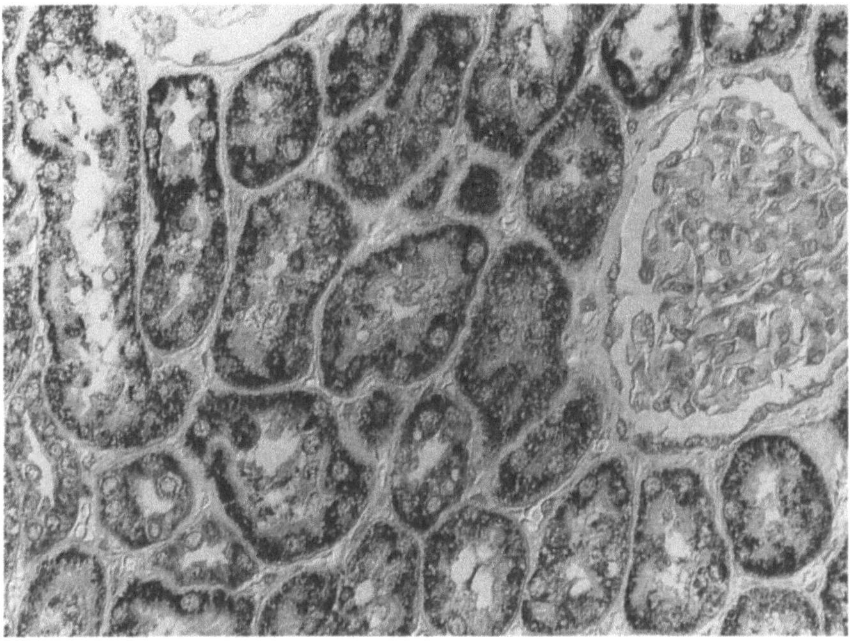

Fig. 5. PTHrP immunoreactivity in the normal adult renal cortex. The immunostaining exhibits a vesicular pattern confined to the tubular epithelium. Polyclonal anti-PTHrP (34–53), avidin-biotin complex technique, nuclear counterstain with hematoxylin, differential interference contrast optics, ×400

showing higher differentiation frequently stained more strongly for PTHrP than did less differentiated areas. A vesicular staining pattern was observed similar to that in normal renal epithelia.

In three cultured renal carcinomas cell lines recently established in our laboratory, PTHrP production was confirmed at both the mRNA and the protein levels. Immunocytochemistry substantiated the hypothesis that the hormone had been packaged into vesicles (Fig. 8). By means of a one-site ELISA for the midregional part, the regulation of PTHrP release into the culture medium was investigated. The secretion is regulated by (1,25)-dihydroxy vitamin D_3, as well as by elevation of extracellular calcium, both of which cause a significant decrease in PTHrP secretion (Fig. 9) in all three cell lines.

The function of PTHrP as an autocrine growth factor in renal cell carcinomas was first observed by Burton et al. (1990a). After specifically blocking the receptor-mediated actions of PTHrP by adding either anti-PTHrP antiserum or a surplus of PTHrP antagonists, a significant decrease in cell proliferation was achieved. Similar results in our cell lines substantiate the role of PTHrP as an autocrine growth factor (Turzynski and Dietel 1993).

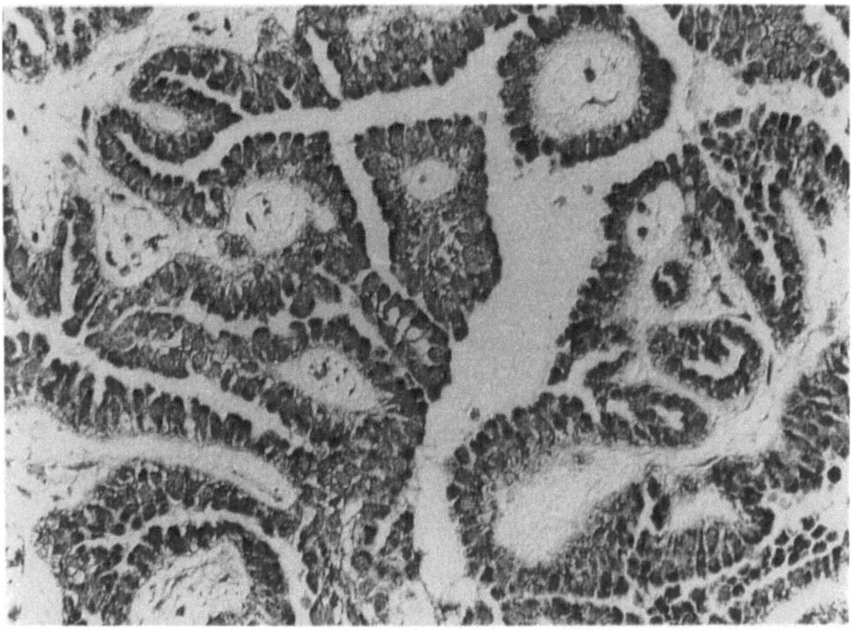

Fig. 6. PTHrP in a renal cell carcinoma. Intense staining in a well-differentiated renal cell carcinoma. Polyclonal anti-PTHrP (34–53), avidin-biotin complex technique, nuclear counterstain with hematoxylin, differential interference contrast optics, ×200

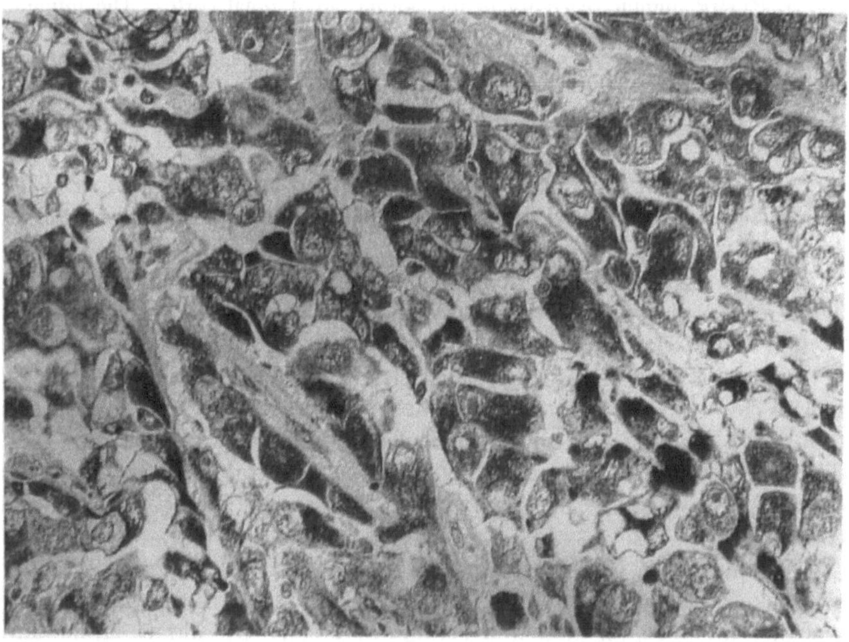

Fig. 7. PTHrP in a renal cell carcinoma. Heteregeneous PTHrP staining pattern in a poorly differentiated renal cell carcinoma. Polyclonal anti-PTHrP (34–53), avidin-biotin complex technique, nuclear counterstain with hematoxylin, differential interference contrast optics, ×400

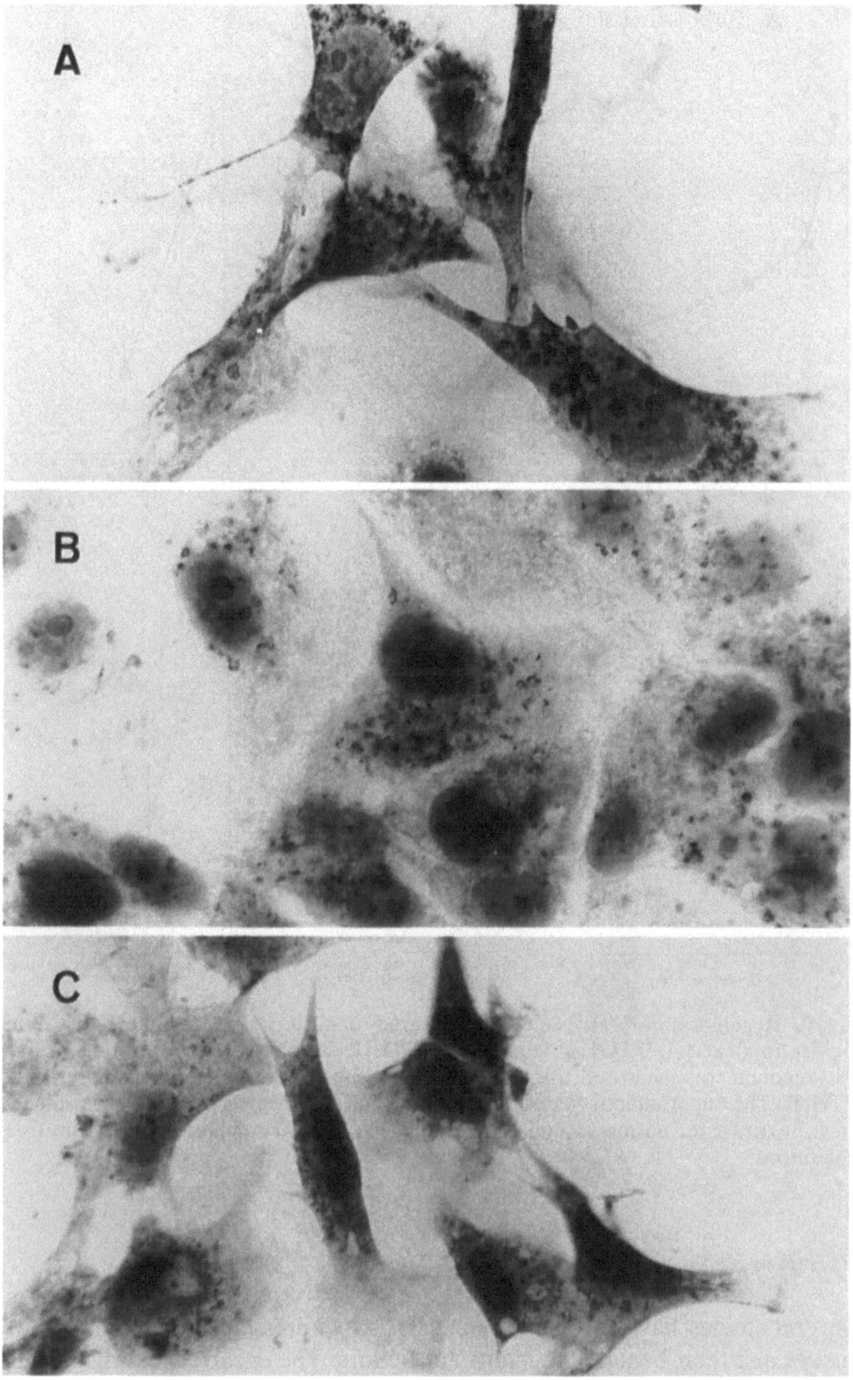

Fig. 8A–C. PTHrP immunoreactivity in three cultured renal carcinoma cell lines RCC 94/92, RCC 95/92, RCC 96/92. PTHrP appears to be packaged in vesicles. Polyclonal anti-PTHrP (34–53), avidin-biotin complex technique, nuclear counterstain with hematoxylin, ×1000

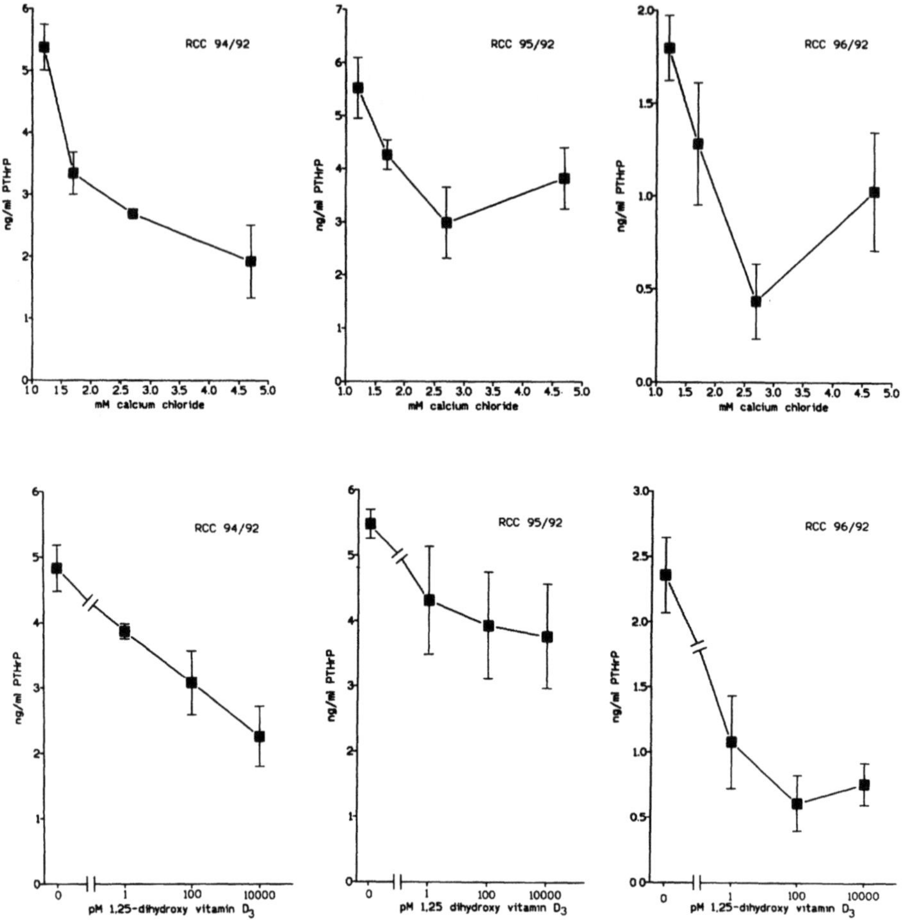

Fig. 9. Regulation of PTHrP release in cultured renal carcinoma cell lines by calcium (*upper row*) and 1,25-$(OH)_2$ vitamin D_3. PTHrP secretion into serum-free Ham's F10 medium was measured using a solid-phase one-site ELISA against midregional PTHrP. The supernatants were harvested after 60 min. Means of three experiments each in triplicate; normocalcemia corresponds to 1.2 m*M* calcium under serum-free conditions

PTHrP in Endocrine Tissues and Their Tumors

Several studies have focussed on the PTHrP expression in neuroendocrine tissues and their benign and malignant tumors. The occurrence of PTHrP in parathyroid glands is of particular interest. In mammalian fetal development relative hypercalcemia compared with maternal serum calcium levels is observed. This might be necessary for the growing skeleton. The fetal-maternal calcium gradient is maintained by a placental calcium pump (Fisher

1986). Following thyroparathyroidectomy in fetal lambs, the plasma calcium concentration decreases below maternal levels (Rodda et al. 1988). The fetal calcium concentration can be restored by PTHrP, but not by PTH. Interestingly, this PTHrP action is not mediated by the common PTH/PTHrP receptor, since the mid-molecular region of PTHrP appears to be the biologically active section for this target. Thus, parathyroid-derived PTHrP serves as the main humoral calcium regulator in fetal development, whereas placental PTHrP and PTH appear to play a minor role, if any.

In adults PTHrP has also been detected in parathyroid glands, by both immunohistochemistry and in situ hybridization (R. Kitizawa et al. 1992). It has even proven possible to clone PTHrP-secreting parathyroid cell lines (Ikeda et al. 1989a). It may be that in this stage PTHrP no longer exerts endocrine effects. In contrast to PTH, the amount of PTHrP that enters the circulation is negligible, and PTHrP secretion in culture sections of bovine parathyroids has been shown to be independent of extracellular calcium levels (Connor et al. 1989). For both these reasons, PTHrP secreted by the parathyroids cannot contribute to the regulation of serum calcium levels in adults.

Here again morphological studies have demonstrated a differentiation or function-dependent localization of PTHrP in parathyroids and their tumors. In normal glands PTHrP was localized by immunohistochemistry and in situ hybidization mainly in the oxyphil cell lineage, especially in transitional cells, and is stored in secretory vesicles (R. Kitizawa et al. 1992). The transitional oxyphil cells contain a well-developed secretory apparatus, and are believed to be derived from the chief cells, whereas typical oxyphil cells are regarded as degenerative.

In parathyroid adenomas, elevated PTHrP immunoreactivity and mRNA can be detected. High PTHrP expression has also been found in parathyroid hyperplasia caused by chronic renal failure. A cytoplasmic vesicular staining pattern has been observed. In contrast, in primary parathyroid hyperplasia PTHrP appears to be clearly absent (Danks et al. 1990). Negative immunostaining was demonstrated by the use of N-terminal, midregional or C-terminal PTHrP antibodies. It is still unknown whether the presence or absence of PTHrP in different disease states is actually biologically significant, whether it is a function of this hormone in the parathyroids, or whether it is only an epiphenomenon.

PTHrP expression has been detected in a variety of other endocrine tissues, such as the anterior lobe of the pituitary gland, the adrenal cortex, the Leydig cells in the testis (Kitazawa et al. 1991), and pancreatic islets (Drucker et al. 1989). If PTHrP expression has biological significance even in these adult endocrine tissues, most likely a local para-/autocrine function of PTHrP must be assumed, although local effects of PTHrP in endocrine tissues have so far not been reported. Nevertheless, PTHrP-mediated hypercalcemia has been attributed to neuroendocrine carcinomas. They include cases of pancreatic islet tumors (Drucker et al. 1989; Mitlak et al. 1991),

Table 1. Sites of production and possible actions of PTHrP. (Modified from Rosol and Capen 1992)

Physiological		Pathological	
- Fetal Parathyroid Glands - Placenta	- Skin - Mammary gland - Kidney - Endocrine tissues - Muscle - Bone - Brain	- Tumors of various origin	- Tumor cell lines
↓	↓	↓	↓
Endocrine	Auto-/paracrine	Endocrine	Autocrine
Calcium homeostasis	Growth and differentiation factor	Humoral hypercalcemia of malignancy	Growth and differentiation factor in tumors

malignant pheochromocytomas, and bronchial carcinoids (Heath et al. 1990). Several endocrine carcinoma cell lines exist that are capable of secreting PTHrP abundantly, such as the Leydig cell carcinoma cell line, the TT cell line derived from a medullary thyroid carcinoma (Ikeda et al. 1989b) and carcinoid tumor cell line (Deftos et al. 1989). In future, they may serve as a valuable tool to elucidate possible functions of PTHrP in neuroendocrine tissues.

Conclusions

The combination of morphological, immunochemical and molecular biological studies on both the RNA and protein levels has revealed a widespread expression of PTHrP in many tissues. Table 1 summarizes the sources of PTHrP and its mode of action. It is either transiently observed during organogenesis and under special developmental circumstances, such as in the lactating mamma, or it is constantly expressed in other tissues. PTHrP is produced by tissues of ecto-, meso-, and entodermal origin and most of them have been shown to secrete this protein in a regulated fashion. It acts by both endocrine and para-/autocrine modes and occurs in both normal and neoplastic tissues. For these reasons, the diversity of possible functions of this effector, e.g., as a calciotropic hormone, a smooth muscle relaxant, a likely neurotransmitter, or a growth and differentiation factor, depends largely on the sites of production and action.

In this perspective the HHM due to PTHrP must be considered most frequently as the result of eutopic hormone production, and consequently appears as the result of changes in the mode of PTHrP actions. It is not yet understood what leads the tumor-derived PTHrP to enter the peripheral circulation, and thus provoke the increase in serum calcium levels. There might be quantitative causes, such as the tumor mass, or there might be qualitative changes in cell function or intercellular communication. Future functional investigations have to clarify the mechanisms of how PTHrP-producing tumors induce HHM.

Acknowledgments. The authors wish to thank B. Schäfer, I. Brand, and P. Neumann for the expert technical assistance and J.P. McFarland for proofreading the paper. This work was supported by the Deutsche Forschungsgemeinschaft, grant no. Di:276/1-5.

References

Atillasoy EJ, Burtis WJ, Milstone LM (1991) Immunohistochemical localization of parathyroid hormone-related protein (PTHRP) in normal human skin. J Invest Dermatol 96:277-280

Barlet JP, Champredon C, Coxam V, Davicco MJ, Tressol JC (1992) Parathyroid hormone-related peptide might stimulate calcium secretion into the milk of goats. J Endocrinol 132:353-359

Berson SA, Yalow RS (1966) Parathyroid hormone in plasma in adenomatous hyperparathyroidism, uremia, and bronchogenic carcinoma. Science 154:907-909

Blind E, Raue F, Götzmann J, Schmidt-Gayk H, Kohl B, Ziegler R (1992) Circulating levels of mid-regional parathyroid hormone-related portein in hypercalcaemia of malignancy. Clin Endocrinol 37:290-297

Bucht E, Carlqvist M, Hedlund B, Bremme K, Torring O (1992) Parathyroid hormone-related peptide in human milk measured by a mid-molecule radioimmunoassay. Metabolism 41:11-16

Budayr AA, Halloran BP, King JC, Diep D, Nissenson RA, Strewler GJ (1989) High levels of a parathyroid hormone-like protein in milk. Proc Natl Acad Sci USA 86:7183-7185

Bundred NJ, Walker RA, Ratcliffe WA, Warwick J, Morrison JM, Ratcliffe JG (1992) Parathyroid hormone related protein and skeletal morbidity in breast cancer. Eur J Cancer 28:690-692

Burtis WJ, Brady TG, Orloff JJ, Ersbak JB, Warrell RP Jr, Olson BR, Wu TL, Mitnick ME, Broadus AE, Stewart AF (1990) Immunochemical characterization of circulating parathyroid hormone-related protein in patients with humoral hypercalcemia of cancer. N Engl J Med 322:1106-1112

Burton PBJ, Knight DE (1992) Parathyroid hormone-related protein can regulate the growth of human lung cancer cells, and may form part of an autocrine TGF-α loop. FEBS Lett 305:228-232

Burton PB, Moniz C, Knight DE (1990a) Parathyroid hormone related peptide can function as an autocrine growth factor in human renal cell carcinoma. Biochem Biophys Res Commun 167:1134-1138

Burton PB, Moniz C, Quirke P, Tzannatos C, Pickles A, Dixit M, Triffit JT, Jueppner H, Segre GV, Knight DE (1990b) Parathyroid hormone-related peptide in the human fetal uro-genital tract. Mol Cell Endocrinol 69:R13-17

Campos RV, Asa SL, Drucker DJ (1991) Immunohistochemical localization of parathyroid hormone-like peptide in the rat fetus. Cancer Res 51:6351-6357

Caulfield MP, McKee RL, Goldman ME, Duong LT, Fisher JE, Gay CT, DeHaven PA, Levy JJ, Roubini E, Nutt RF et al. (1990) The bovine renal parathyroid hormone (PTH) receptor has equal affinity for two different amino acid sequences: the receptor binding domains of PTH and PTH-related protein are located within the 14–34 region. Endocrinology 127:83–87

Connor CS, Drees BM, Thurston A, Forte L, Hermreck AS, Hamilton JVV (1989) Bovine parathyroid tissue: a model to compare the biosynthesis and secretion of parathyroid hormone and parathyroid hormone-related peptide. Surgery 106: 1057–1062

Danks JA, Ebeling PR, Hayman J, Chou ST, Moseley JM, Dunlop J, Kemp BE, Martin TJ (1989) Parathyroid hormone-related protein: immunohistochemical localization in cancers and in normal skin. J Bone Miner Res 4:273–278

Danks JA, Ebeling PR, Hayman JA, Diefenbach-Jagger H, Collier FM, Grill V, Southby J, Moseley JM, Chou ST, Martin TJ (1990) Immunohistochemical localization of parathyroid hormone-related protein in parathyroid adenoma and hyperplasia. J Pathol 161:27–33

Deftos LJ, Gazdar AF, Ikeda K, Broadus AE (1989) The parathyroid hormone-related protein associated with malignancy is secreted by neuroendocrine tumors. Mol Endocrinol 3:503–508

Dietel M, Dorn-Quint G (1980) By-pass secretion of human parathyroid adenomas. Lab Invest 43:116–125

Drucker DJ, Asa SL, Henderson J, Goltzman D (1989) The parathyroid hormone-like peptide gene is expressed in the normal and neoplastic human endocrine pancreas. Mol Endocrinol 3:1589–1595

Ellis AG, Adam WR, Martin TJ (1990) Comparison of the effects of parathyroid hormone (PTH) and recombinant PTH-related protein on bicarbonate excretion by the isolated perfused rat kidney. J Endocrinol 126:403–408

Ellison M, Woodhouse D, Hillyard CJ, Dowsett M, Coombes RC, Gilby ED, Greenberg PB, Neville AM (1975) Immunoreactive calcitonin production by human lung carcinoma cells in culture. Br J Cancer 32:373–379

Ferrari SL, Rizzoli R, Bonjour JP (1992) Parathyroid hormone-related protein production by primary cultures of mammary epithelial cells. J Cell Physiol 150: 304–311

Fisher DA (1986) The unique endocrine milieu of the fetus. J Clin Invest 78:603–611

Grill V, Ho P, Body JJ, Johanson N, Lee SC, Kukreja SC, Moseley JM, Martin TJ (1991) Parathyroid hormone-related protein: elevated levels in both humoral hypercalcemia of malignancy and hypercalcemia complicating metastatic breast cancer. J Clin Endocrinol Metab 73:1309–1315

Gupta A, Martin KJ, Miyauchi A, Hruska KA (1991) Regulation of cytosolic calcium by parathyroid hormone and oscillations of cytosolic calcium in fibroblasts from normal and pseudohypoparathyroid patients. Endocrinology 128:2825–2836

Hayman JA, Danks JA, Ebeling PR, Moseley JM, Kemp BE, Martin TJ (1989) Expression of parathyroid hormone related protein in normal skin and in tumours of skin and skin appendages. J Pathol 158:293–296

Heath DA, Senior PV, Varley JM, Beck F (1990) Parathyroid-hormone-related protein in tumours associated with hypercalcaemia. Lancet 335:66–69

Henderson JE, Shustik C, Kremer R, Rabbani SA, Hendy GN, Goltzman D (1990) Circulating concentrations of parathyroid hormone-like peptide in malignancy and in hyperparathyroidism. J Bone Miner Rse 5:105–113

Hoekman K, Lowik CW, v.d. Ruit M, Kempenaar J, Bijvoet OL, Ponec M (1990) Modulation of the production of a parathyroid hormone-like protein in human squamous carcinoma cell lines by interaction with fibroblasts. Cancer Res 50: 3589–3594

Holick MF, Nussbaum S, Persons KS (1988) PTH-like humeral hypercalcemia factor (HHF) of malignancy may be an epidermal differentiation factor: synthetic hHHF

(1–34)NH_2 inhibits proliferation and induces terminal differentiation of cultured human keratinocytes (abstract 582). J Bone Mineral Res 3[Suppl]:214
Ikeda K, Weir EC, Sakaguchi K, Burtis WJ, Zimering M, Mangin M, Dreyer BE, Brandi ML, Aurbach GD, Broadus AE (1989a) Clonal rat parathyroid cell line expresses a parathyroid hormone-related peptide but not parathyroid hormone itself. Biochem Biophys Res Comm 162:108–115
Ikeda K, Lu C, Weir EC, Mangin M, Broadus AE (1989b) Transcriptional regulation of the parathyroid hormone-related peptide gene by glucocorticoids and vitamin D in a human C-cell line. J Biol Chem 264:15743–15746
Ivell R (1993) The detection of neuropeptide mRNA in the testis is not evidence for local biosynthesis of the hormones (abstract). Exp Clin Endocrinol 101:97
Jüppner H, Abou Samra AB, Freeman M, Kong XF, Schipani E, Richards J, Kolakowski LF Jr, Hock J, Potts JT Jr, Kronenberg HM, Segre GV (1991) A G protein-linked receptor for parathyroid hormone and parathyroid hormone-related peptide. Science 254:1024–1026
Kao PC, Klee GG, Taylor RL, Heath H 3d (1990) Parathyroid hormone-related peptide in plasma of patients with hypercalcemia and malignant lesions. Mayo Clin Proc 65:1399–1407
Kitazawa R, Kitazawa S, Fukase M, Fujita T, Kobayashi A, Chihara K, Maeda S (1992) The expression of parathyroid hormone-related protein (PTHrP) in normal parathyroid: histochemistry and in situ hybridization. Histochemistry 98:211–215
Kitazawa S, Fukase M, Kitazawa R, Takenaka A, Gotoh A, Fujita T, Maeda S (1991) Immunohistologic evaluation of parathyroid hormone-related protein in human lung cancer and normal tissue with newly developed monoclonal antibody. Cancer 67:984–989
Kitazawa S, Kitazawa R, Fukase M, Fujimori T, Maeda S (1992) Immunohistochemical evaluation of parathyroid hormone-related protein (PTHrP) in the uterine cervix. Int J Cancer 50:731–735
Koji T, Brenner RM (1993) Localization of estrogen receptor messenger ribonucleic acid in rhesus monkey uterus by nonradioactive in situ hybridization with digoxigenin-labeled oligodeoxynucleotides. Endocrinology 132:382–392
le Guellec P, Dumas S, Volle GE, Pidoux E, Moukhtar MS, Treilhou-Lahille F (1993) An efficient method to detect calcitonin mRNA in normal and neoplastic rat C-cells (medullary thyroid carcinoma) by in situ hybridization using a digoxigenin-labeled synthetic oligodeoxyribonucleotide probe. J Histochem Cytochem 41:389–395
Lin HY, Harris TL, Flannery MS, Aruffo A, Kaji EH, Gorn A, Kolakowski LF Jr, Lodish HF, Goldring SR (1991) Expression cloning of an adenylate cyclase-coupled calcitonin receptor. Science 254:1022–1024
Mangin M, Ikeda K, Dreyer BE, Milstone L, Broadus AE (1988) Two distinct tumor-derived, parathyroid hormone-like peptides result from alternative ribonucleic acid splicing. Mol Endocrinol 2:1049–1055
Martin TJ, Allan EH, Caple JW, Care AD, Danks JA, Diefenbach-Jagger H, Ebeling PR, Gillespie MT, Hammonds G, Heath JA, Hudson PJ, Kemp BE, Kubota M, Kukreja SC, Moseley JM, Ng KW, Raisz LG, Rodda CP, Simmons HA, Suva LJ, Wettenhall REH, Woods WI (1989) Parathyroid hormone-related protein: isolation, molecular cloning, and mechanism of action. Recent Prog Horm Res 45:467–502
Merendino TJ, Insogna KL, Milstone LM, Broadus AE, Stewart AF (1986) Parathyroid hormone-like protein from cultured human keratinocytes. Science 231:388–390
Mitlak BH, Hutchison JS, Kaufman SD, Nussbaum SR (1991) Parathyroid hormone-related peptide mediates hypercalcemia in an islet cell tumor of the pancreas. Horm Metab Res 23:344–346

Moniz C, Burton PB, Malik AN, Dixit M, Banga JP, Nicolaides K, Quirke P, Knight DE, McGregor AM (1990) Parathyroid hormone-related peptide in normal human fetal development. J Mol Endocrinol 5:259–266

Moseley JM, Kubota M, Diefenbach-Jagger H, Wettenhall REH, Kemp BE, Suva LJ, Rodda CP, Ebeling PR, Hudson PJ, Zajac JD, Martin TJ (1987) Parathyroid hormone-related protein purified from a human lung cancer cell line. Proc Natl Acad Sci USA 84:5048–5052

Musso MJ, Plante M, Judes C, Barthelmebs M, Helwig JJ (1989) Renal vasodilatation and microvessel adenylate cyclase stimulation by synthetic parathyroid hormone-like protein fragments. Eur J Pharmacol 174:139–151

Mussbaum SR, Gaz RD, Arnold A (1990) Hypercalcemia and ectopic secretion of parathyroid hormone by an ovarian carcinoma with rearrangement of the gene for parathyroid hormone. N Engl J Med 323:1324–1328

Orloff JJ, Ganz MB, Ribaudo AE, Burtis WJ, Reiss M, Milstone LM, Stewart AF (1992) Analysis of PTHRP binding and signal transduction mechanisms in benign and malignant squamous cells. Am J Physiol 262:E599–607

Pizurki L, Rizzoli R, Moseley J, Martin TJ, Caverzasio J, Bonjour JP (1988) Effect of synthetic tumoral PTH-related peptide on cAMP production and Na-dependent Pi transport. Am J Physiol 255:F957–961

Powell GJ, Southby J, Danks JA, Stillwell RG, Hayman JA, Henderson MA, Bennett RC, Martin TJ (1991) Localization of parathyroid hormone-related protein in breast cancer metastases: increased incidence in bone compared with other sites. Cancer Res 51:3059–3061

Ralston SH, Danks J, Hayman J, Fraqser D, Stewart CS, Martin TJ (1991) Parathyroid hormone-related protein of malignancy: immunohistochemical and biochemical studies in normocalcaemic and hypercalcaemic patients with cancer. J Clin Pathol 44:472–476

Rodda CP, Kubota M, Heath JA, Ebeling PR, Moseley JM, Care AD, Caple IW, Martin TJ (1988) Evidence for a novel parathyroid hormone-related protein in fetal lamb parathyroid glands and sheep placenta: comparisons with a similar protein implicated in humoral hypercalcaemia of malignancy. J Endocrinol 117: 261–271

Rosol TJ, Capen CC (1992) Biology of disease. Mechanisms of cancer-induced hypercalcemia. Lab Invest 67:680–702

Selvanayagam P, Graves K, Cooper C, Rajaraman S (1991) Expression of the parathyroid hormone-related peptide gene in rat tissues. Lab Invest 64:713–717

Shorrock K, Roberts P, Pringle JH, Lauder I (1991) Demonstration of insulin and glucagon mRNA in routinely fixed and processed pancreatic tissue by in-situ hybridization. J Pathol 165:105–110

Southby J, Kissin MW, Danks JA, Hayman JA, Moseley JM, Henderson MA, Bennett RC, Martin TJ (1990) Immunohistochemical localization of parathyroid hormone-related protein in human breast cancer. Cancer Res 50:7710–7716

Suva LJ, Mather KA, Gillespie MT, Webb GC, Ng KW, Winslow GA, Wood WI, Martin TJ, HudsonPJ (1989) Structure of the 5′ flanking region of the gene encoding human parathyroid-hormone-related protein (PTHrP). Gene 77:95–105

Tachimori Y, Watanabe H, Kato H, Yamaguchi H, Nagasaki K, Honda S, Itabashi M, Yamaguchi K (1991) Hypercalcemia in patients with esophageal carcinoma. The pathophysiologic role of parathyroid hormone-related protein. Cancer 68: 2625–2629

Thiede MA (1989) The mRNA encoding a parathyroid hormone-like peptide is produced in mammary tissue in response to elevations in serum prolactin. Mol Endocrinol 3:1443–1447

Thiede MA, Strewler GJ, Nissenson RA, Rosenblatt M, Rodan GA (1988) Human renal carcinoma expresses two messages encoding a parathyroid hormone-like

peptide: evidence for the alternative splicing of a single copy gene. Proc Natl Acad Sci USA 85:4605–4609
Turzynski A, Dietel M (1993) Parathyroid hormone-related protein (PTHrP) – an autocrine stimulator of proliferation in renal carcinoma cell lines (abstract). Exp Clin Endocrinol 101:175
Wu TL, Soifer NE, Burtis WJ, Milstone LM, Stewart AF (1991) Glycosylation of parathyroid hormone-related peptide secreted by human epidermal keratinocytes. J Clin Endocrinol Metab 73:1002–1007
Yamamoto M, Fisher JE, Thiede MA, Caulfield MP, Rosenblatt M, Duong LT (1992) Concentrations of parathyroid hormone-related protein in rat milk change with duration of lactation and interval from previous suckling, but not with milk calcium. Endocrinology 130:741–747
Yoshimoto K, Yamasaki R, Sakai H, Tezuka U, Takahashi M, Iizuka, Sekiya T, Saito S (1989) Ectopic production of parathyroid hormone by small cell lung cancer in a patient with hypercalcemia. J Clin Endocrinol Metab 68:976–981
Zhou H, Leaver DD, Moseley JM, Kemp B, Ebeling PR, Martin TJ (1989) Actions of parathyroid hormone-related protein on the rat kidney in vivo. J Endocrinol 122:229–235

Clinical Aspects

Epidemiological Aspects of Hypercalcemia of Malignancy

F. Raue

Department of Internal Medicine I – Endocrinology and Metabolism, University of Heidelberg, Bergheimerstraße 58, 69115 Heidelberg, Germany

Hypercalcemia can be caused by many disorders, but is most commonly due to primary hyperparathyroidism and to malignant disease. Together, these account for more than 90% of all cases. Many patients with primary hyperparathyroidism are asymptomatic and ambulant when hypercalcemia is first recognized by routine measurement of serum calcium levels. However, the incidence of hypercalcemia of cancer, which has been estimated to be about 150 new cases per million persons per year, is not as high as the annual incidence rate of primary hyperparathyroidism (approximately 250 new cases per year) (Burkhardt and Kistler 1981; Heath et al. 1980; Mundy et al. 1980, 1984).

Hypercalcemia is the most common life-threatening metabolic disorder associated with cancer. It has been estimated that hypercalcemia occurs in 10%–20% of cancer patients at some time during the course of the disease (Burt and Brennan 1980; Myers 1973). When hypercalcemia results from malignancy the cancer is rarely occult, and the clinical features differ from those of primary hyperparathyroidism. Hypercalcemia secondary to cancer is usually steadily progressive, and the patient may experience symptoms despite a relatively low concentration of serum calcium. Typical clinical features of primary hyperparathyroidism, such as renal calculi, are much less common in cancer, probably because hypercalciuria and hypercalcemia are of shorter duration (Blind et al. 1990). Psychiatric and neurologic symptoms related to hypercalcemia such as nausea, vomiting, anorexia, lethargy, confusion, stupor and sometimes coma occur more often and may be easily mistaken for the terminal features of cancer or the side effects of cancer chemotherapy or radiotherapy.

The incidence of hypercalcemia varies depending on the type of cancer. This variability is due presumably to differences in the mediating factors, including parathyroid hormone related protein (PTHrP), and clinical circumstances, e.g., osteolytic metastases, responsible for the onset of hypercalcemia (Muggia 1990). For example, patients with carcinomas of the breast, lung, head and neck, and those with certain hematologic malignancies, e.g., multiple myeloma, have a higher incidence of associated hypercalcemia, whereas hypercalcemia is rare in patients with carcinoma of the colon. Most patients with hypercalcemia of malignancy have evidence of distant metastases, often to bone, but in the remaining minority tumor deposits in bone cannot be demonstrated. It is in the latter group in particular that humoral mediators of cancer-related hypercalcemia are involved, including PTHrP, transforming growth factor α (TGFα), and cytokines such as interleukin 1 (IL-1) and tumor necrosis factor (TNF) (Bertolini et al. 1986; Gowen et al. 1983; Rosol and Capen 1992).

Malignant Status Associated with Hypercalcemia

In cancer patients and hospitalized patients in general, malignancy is the most common cause of hypercalcemia but other causes have to be excluded. The importance of a carefully executed differential diagnostic workup in cancer patients is illustrated by the finding that in hospitalized cancer patients only 77% of hypercalcemia cases were caused by the malignancy itself; 4% of the cancer patients had coexistent primary hyperparathyroidism, 2% had vitamin D intoxication, 2% had tamoxifen-induced hypercalcemia and in 16% the cancer was attributed to an idiopathic etiology (Blomqvist 1986). A differential diagnosis is essential in cancer patients with hypercalcemia so that therapy can be directed toward the underlying pathogenetic mechanisms.

Hypercalcemia has been reported to affect approximately 20% of all patients with cancer at some time during the course of the disease (Myers 1973). The likelihood that cancer patients will have a higher calcium level will be influenced by the duration of illness or survival and the frequency of testing. The reported prevalence of hypercalcemia reflects data accumulated from patients observed over many years. In a study from the M.D. Anderson Cancer Center, the incidence of hypercalcemia was relatively low in patients with malignant disease, only 1.1% (88 out of 7667 patients in 1 year) (Vassilopoulou-Sellin et al. 1993), but higher than the incidence reported by Mundy et al. 1980 (0.07%). This can probably be attributed to the referral patterns of a large cancer center. Similar incidence data from patients in hospital were reported by Fisken et al. (1981), Ralston et al. (1990), Blind et al. (1990) and Blomqvist (1986).

The relative frequency of the different primary cancer sites that are associated with hypercalcemia is presented in Table 1. The most common causes of hypercalcemia are cancers of the lung and breast, which accounted for 22%–60% of the total series (Blind et al. 1990; Blomqvist 1986; Fisken et al. 1980; Ralston et al. 1990; Stewart et al. 1988). Among lung cancers, hypercalcemia is most commonly associated with squamous cell tumors and rarely with small cell cancer of the lung. Some common cancers are seldom complicated by hypercalcemia, including colorectal cancers and prostate

Table 1. Relative frequency of different types of malignancy associated with hypercalcemia

Primary site of cancer	Percentage of cases				
	Fisken et al. (1980)	Blomqvist (1986)	Stewart et al. (1988)	Ralston et al. (1990)	Blind et al. (1990)
Lung	25	28	35	34	7
Breast	20	39	25	17	15
Hematologic (myeloma, lymphoma)	11	13	14	10	31
Head and neck	7	6	6	4	8
Genitourinary	18	6	6	12	17

cancer. On the other hand, several relatively uncommon cancers are frequently associated with hypercalcemia; these include cholangiocarcinoma and clear cell carcinoma of the ovary. Hematologic malignancies can be complicated by hypercalcemia. Up to one-third of patients with myeloma have complicating hypercalcemia, but because of its relative rarity this type of cancer does not significantly influence most reported series. Association of specific cancers with hypercalcemia is presumably related to the capacity of these tumors to secrete specific factors which induce hypercalcemia and/or metastases of bone. It is striking that primary bone tumors, e.g., osteogenic sarcoma, virtually never cause hypercalcemia.

The majority of patients with hypercalcemia of malignancy have obvious widespread metastases at the time hypercalcemia is diagnosed; for example, 86% of patients with solid tumors had obvious metastatic disease (Blomqvist 1986). Only a very few of these patients have a tumor that is curable by primary resection. In a review of the world literature 64 cases were found in which removal of the tumor corrected the hypercalcemia (Skrabanek et al. 1980). As hypercalcemia is usually a manifestation of advanced malignancy it is rare for it to present before a stage at which a curable resection of the tumor is possible. In a systematic evaluation of hypercalcemia in patients with cancer attending a large oncology center, it was noted that the mean latency time between primary diagnosis of the tumor and detection of hypercalcemia was 26 months (Blomqvist 1986).

The prognosis of patients with cancer-associated hypercalcemia is remarkably poor: In one study 50% of the patients died within 1 month and nearly 75% died within 3 months of starting antihypercalcemic therapy (Ralston et al. 1990). Survival was even shorter in the study by Warrell et al. (1988), in which the actual median survival was only 29 days. By comparison, Mundy and Martin (1982) reported that most patients with cancer-associated hypercalcemia survived from 3 to 6 months from presentation, and in the studies of Fisken et al. (1980) and Blomquist (1986) median survival was between 2 and 3 months. The poor prognosis might be due to death from hypercalcemic crisis or to the fact that the development of hypercalcemia is simply a marker of advanced disease. In a study of 218 patients with renal cell carcinomas the incidence of hypercalcemia increased with the tumor stage: 3% stage I, 5.9% stage II, 14.1% stage III, 18.9% stage IV (Fahn et al. 1991). Although the presence of hypercalcemia was indicative of a large tumor burden or a dire prognosis, survival curves between hypercalcemic and eucalcemic patients with stage I–III disease were not significantly different. But in stage IV cancer patients hypercalcemia was associated with a significant deterioration in survival: 45 days in hypercalcemic and 286 days in eucalcemic patients. In the study by Ralston et al. (1990), most patients treated with antihypercalcemic therapy in conjunction with a specific anticancer therapy died from progressive cancer or its complications, with normal or only slightly elevated serum calcium levels before death. Following antihypercalcemic therapy in patients with cancer, symptoms of hypercalcemia markedly improved but without an effect on survival. Thus, antihypercalcemic therapy is a palliative measure that should probably be reserved for patients with symptoms.

Hypercalcemia associated with solid tumors which may or may not be accompanied by bone metastases, e.g., lung, renal, and ovarian cancer, is usually called humoral hypercalcemia of malignancy. The second type of hypercalcemia is associated with solid tumors which are accompanied by extensive bone metastases. Hypercalcemia in these patients is due to bone destruction caused by the metastatic process. The most frequent example in this group is breast cancer. The third type of hypercalcemia is associated hematologic malignancy; here, hypercalcemia seems to be due to a combination of increased bone resorption and increased absorption of calcium from the gut or impaired glomerular filtration (i.e., as in multiple myeloma) (Muggia 1990; Mundy 1990; Mundy et al. 1984).

Hypercalcemia Associated with Specific Neoplastic Conditions

Carcinoma of the Lung

It has been well demonstrated that hypercalcemia occurs most typically with squamous cell carcinoma of the lung despite the fact that adenocarcinoma and small cell carcinoma more frequently metastasize to bone (Bender and Hansen 1974). The incidence of hypercalcemia in lung cancer is about 12%–35% (Fisken et al. 1980; Mundy and Martin 1982). A retrospective review by Coggeshall et al. (Coggeshall et al. 1986; Mundy and Martin 1982) of 67 patients with lung cancer and hypercalcemia found that none of the patients presented with surgically curable lung cancer. Hypercalcemia was always associated with large tumor masses. Although the disease is often disseminated, bone metastases are not necessarily present and there is no correlation between the presence of metastases and hypercalcemia. The median survival time after development of hypercalcemia as a complication of carcinoma of the lung was 1 month (range 1 week to 10 months).

Breast Cancer

The term "breast cancer" encompasses a category of malignant disease that accounts for about 25% of all patients with hypercalcemia of malignancy (Mundy and Martin 1982). Hypercalcemia occurs during the course of the disease in 30%–40% of patients with malignant tumors of the breast (Galasko and Burn 1971; Hickey et al. 1981). The incidence of bone destruction caused by metastatic disease varies greatly but occurs in approximately two-thirds of patients (Coleman and Rubens 1987; Scheid et al. 1986). Reports of hypercalcemia occurring in breast cancer patients in the absence of bone metastases (Isales et al. 1987) and the observation that some patients with extensive metastases may not develop hypercalcemia suggest that in some patients bone destruction is mediated by humoral factors and is not due only to bone destruction caused by metastatic processes. One of these humoral factors is PTHrP; it was detectable in the plasma of 92% of hypercalcemic patients with bone metastases compared with 36% of normocalcemic patients with bone metastases and 9% of normocalcemic patients without bone metastases (Bundred et al. 1991). Tumor-derived PTHrP may have an important humoral role in hypercalcemia associated with metastatic breast cancer. PTHrP was localized by immunohistology in 92% of breast cancer metastases in bone and in 17% of metastases in non-bone sites (Powell et al. 1991). PTHrP positivity in the primary tumor was related to the development of bone metastases and hypercalcemic episodes in the follow-up (Bundred et al. 1992). If PTHrP production by primary tumors provides a means of identifying those at risk for development of bone involvement, it would allow selection of those most likely to benefit from specific treatments aimed at preventing bone metastases, e.g., bisphosphonates (Elomaa et al. 1983). Hypercalcemia may occur after hormone therapy, i.e., estrogens, androgens, progestins or tamoxifen (Coleman et al. 1988; Legha et al. 1981; Mundy 1988; Otteman and Long 1984). Rarely is the cause of severe hypercalcemia, with or without metastases, coexisting primary hyperparathyroidism (Hickey et al. 1981). Approximately 90% of patients dying with breast cancer have bone metastases (Galasko 1971; Sklaroff 1968) and their median survival after diagnosis of hypercalcemia is about 3 months (Coleman and Rubens 1985).

Hematologic Malignancies

Hypercalcemia has always been recognized as a common complication of myeloma but has been thought to be a rather rare, late complication in the leukemias and lymphomas; however, it is common in HTLV-1 associated T-cell lymphoma (Bunn et al. 1983; Grossmann 1981). Virtually all patients with multiple myeloma have extensive osteolytic bone destruction and approximately 20%–40% of patients with myeloma develop hypercalcemia at some time during the course of their disease (Burt and Brennan 1980; Fisken et al. 1980; Kyle 1985). For many patients hypercalcemia is part of the terminal development of the myeloma (Buckman et al. 1982; Durie and Salmon 1982). Hypercalcemia may be expected whenever patients become bedridden and may cause or contribute to renal failure. Hypercalcemia in myeloma always occurs in the presence of extensive bone destruction occurring adjacent to collections of myeloma cells. Bone resorption is caused by the release of several cytokines including IL-1, lymphotoxin, and TNF, each of which has been identified as a potent stimulator of osteoclastic bone resorption in vitro (Bertolini et al. 1986; Gowen et al. 1983). In some lymphomas, PTHrP and 1,25$(OH)_2$ vitamin D may be involved (Breslau et al. 1984; McCanley et al. 1992).

References

Bender RA, Hansen H (1974) Hypercalcemia in bronchogenic carcinoma: a prospective study of 200 patients. Ann Intern Med 80:205–208

Bertolini DR, Nedwin GE, Bringman TS, Mundy GR (1986) Stimulation of bone resorption and inhibition of bone formation in vitro by human tumor necrosis factor. Nature 319:515–518

Blind E, Raue F, Zisterer A, Kohl B, Ziegler R (1990) Epidemiologie der Hypercalcämie, Bedeutung der Bestimmung des intakten Parathormons für die Differentialdiagnose. Dtsch Med Wochenschr 115:1739–1745

Blomqvist CP (1986) Malignant hypercalcemia: a hospital survey. Acta Med Scand 220:455–463

Breslau NA, McGuire JL, Zerwekh JE, Frenkel EP, Pak CYC (1984) Hypercalcemia associated with increased serum calcitriol levels in three patients with lymphoma. Ann Intern Med 100:1–7

Buckman R, Cuzick J, Galton DAG (1982) Long term survival in myelomatosis: a report to the MRC working party on leukaemia in adults. Br J Haematol 52: 589–559

Bundred NJ, Ratcliffe WA, Walker RA, Coley S, Morrison JM, Ratcliffe JR (1991) Parathyroid hormone related protein and hypercalcemia in breast cancer. Br J Cancer 303:1506–1509

Bundred NJ, Walker RA, Ratcliffe WA, Warwick J, Morrison JM, Ratcliffe JR (1992) Parathyroid hormone-related protein and skeletal morbidity in breast cancer. Eur J Cancer 28:690–692

Bunn PA, Schlechter GP, Jaffe E, Blayney D, Young RC, Matthew MJ, Blattner W, Broder S, Gadroff MR, Gallo RC (1983) Clinical course of retrovirus-associated adult T-cell lymphoma in the US. N Engl J Med 309:257–264

Burkhardt E, Kistler JJ (1981) Hypercalciämie bei hospitalisierten Patienten. Schweiz Med Wochenschr 111:2017–2023

Burt ME, Brennan MF (1980) Incidence of hypercalcemia and malignant neoplasm. Arch Surg 115:704–707

Coggeshall J, Merrill W, Hande K, Prez RD (1986) Implications of hypercalcemia with respect to diagnosis and treatment of lung cancer. Am J Med 80:325–328
Coleman RE, Rubens RD (1985) Bone metastases and breast cancer. Cancer Treat Rev. 12:251–270
Coleman RE, Rubens RD (1987) The clinical course of bone metastases from breast cancer. Br J Cancer 55:61–66
Coleman RL, Fogelman I, Rubens RD (1988) Hypercalcemia and breast cancer: an increased humoral component in patients with liver metastases. Eur J Surg Oncol 14:428–443
Durie BGM, Salmon SE (1982) Current status and future prospects for treatment in multiple myeloma. Clin Haematol 11:181–210
Elomaa I, Blomquist C, Grohn P, Porkka L, Kairento AL, Selander K, Lamberg-Allardt G, Holmstrom T (1983) Long-term controlled trial with diphosphonate in patients with osteologic bone metastases. Lancet i:146–148
Fahn HJ, Lee YH, Chen MT, Huang JK, Chen KK, Chang LS (1991) The incidence and prognostic significance of humoral hypercalcemia in renal cell carcinoma. J Urol 145:248–250
Fisken RA, Heath DA, Bold AM (1980) Hypercalcemia – a hospital survey. Q J Med 49:405–418
Fisken RA, Heath DA, Somers S (1981) Hypercalcemia in hospital patients: clinical and diagnostic aspects. Lancet i:202–207
Galasko CSB, Burn JL (1971) Hypercalcemia in patients with advanced mammary cancer. Br Med J 3:573–577
Gowen M, Wood OD, Ihrie EJ, McGuire MKB, Russell RGG (1983) An interleukin 1 like factor stimulates bone resorption in vitro. Nature 306:376–380
Grossmann B, Schechter GP, Horton JE, Pierce L, Juffe E, Wahl L (1981) Hypercalcemia associated with T-cell lymphoma-leukemia. Am J Clin Pathol 75: 149–155
Heath H III, Hodgson SF, Kennedy MA (1980) Primary hyperparathyroidism: incidence, morbidity, and potential economic impact in a community. N Engl J Med 302:189–193
Hickey RC, Samaan NA, Jackson GL (1981) Hypercalcemia in patients with breast cancer. Arch Surg 116:545–552
Isales C, Carangiu ML, Stewart AF (1987) Hypercalcemia in breast cancer: reassessment of the mechanism. Am J Med 82:1142–1147
Kyle RA (1985) Multiple myeloma: current therapy and a glimpse of the future. Scand J Haematol 35:38–47
Legha SS, Powell K, Buzdar AU, Blumenschein GR (1981) Tamoxifen-induced hypercalcemia in breast cancer. Cancer 47:2803–2806
McCanley LK, Rosol TJ, Merryman JI, Capen CC (1992) Parathyroid hormone-related protein binding to human T-cell lymphotropic virus type I-infected lymphocytes. Endocrinology 130:300–306
Muggia FM (1990) Overview of cancer-related hypercalcemia: epidemiology and etiology. Semin Oncol 17[Suppl 5]:3–9
Mundy GR (1988) Hypercalcemia of malignancy revisited. J Clin Invest 82:1–6
Mundy GR (1990) Pathophysiology of cancer-associated hypercalcemia. Semin Oncol 17[Suppl 5]:10–15
Mundy GR, Martin TJ (1982) The hypercalcemia of malignancy: pathogenesis and management. Metabolism 31:1247–1277
Mundy GR, Cove DH, Fisken R (1980) Primary hyperparathyroidism: changes in the pattern of clinical presentation. Lancet i:1317–1320
Mundy GR, Ibbotson KJ, D'Souza SM, Simpson EL, Jacobs JW, Martin TJ (1984) The hypercalcemia of cancer: clinical implications and pathologic mechanisms. N Engl J Med 310:1718–1727

Myers WPL (1973) Hypercalcemia associated with maligant diseases. In: Schwartz TB (ed) Endocrine and nonendocrine hormone-producing tumors. Year Book Medical Publishers, Chicago, pp 147–171

Otteman LA, Long HJ (1984) Hypercalcemic flare with megestol acetate. Cancer Treat Rep 68:1420–1421

Powell GJ, Southby J, Danks JA, Stillwell RG, Hayman JA, Henderson MA, Bennett RC, Martin TJ (1991) Localization of parathyroid hormone-related protein in breast cancer metastases: increased incidence in bone compared with other sites. Cancer Res 51:3059–3061

Ralston SH, Gallagher SJ, Patel U, Campbell J, Boyle IT (1990) Cancer-associated hypercalcemia: morbidity and mortality clinical experience in 126 treated patients. Ann Intern Med 112:499–504

Rosol TJ, Capen CC (1992) Biology of disease: mechanisms of cancer-induced hypercalcemia. Lab Invest 67:680–702

Scheid V, Buzdar AU, Smith TL, Hortobagyi GN (1986) Clinical course of breast cancer patients with osseous metastases treated with combination chemotherapy. Cancer 58:2589–2593

Sklaroff DM, Charker ND (1968) Bone metastases from breast cancer at the time of the radical mastectomy. Surg Gynecol Obstet 127:763–768

Skrabanek P, McPartlin M, Powell D (1980) Tumor hypercalcemia and "ectopic hyperparathyroidism". Medicine 59:262–282

Stewart AF, Mangin M, Wu T, Goumas D, Insogna KL, Burtis WJ, Broadus AE (1988) Synthetic human parathyroid hormone-like protein stimulates bone resorption and causes hypercalcemia in rats. J Clin Invest 81:596–600

Vassilopoulou-Sellin R, Newman BM, Taylor SH, Guinee VF (1993) Incidence of hypercalcemia in patients with malignancy referred to a comprehensive cancer center. Cancer 71:1309–1312

Warrell RP, Israel R, Frisone M, Snyder T, Gaynor JJ, Bockman RS (1988) Gallium nitrate for acute treatment of cancer-related hypercalcemia: a randomized, double-lind comparison to calcitonin. Ann Intern Med 108:669–674

Clinical Picture of Humoral Hypercalcemia of Malignancy

R. Ziegler

Department of Internal Medicine I – Endocrinology and Metabolism, University of Heidelberg, Bergheimerstraße 58, 69115 Heidelberg, Germany

Hypercalcemic Syndrome

Hypercalcemia is generally the symptom of a disease which requires treatment. Only in rare conditions such as hypocalciuric hypercalcemia or truly asymptomatic, nonprogressive primary hyperparathyroidism is observation of hypercalcemia without treatment justified. In such cases, hypercalcemia is mild. Severely elevated plasma levels regardless of the underlying disease cause symptoms which are summarized as the "hypercalcemic syndrome" (Table 1). All such symptoms are functional and can be reversed by lowering calcium levels to normal. Single symptoms are not enough to diagnose a disease, but the more disturbances that are present in the patient, the more a plasma calcium determination is necessary to exclude hypercalcemia. Hypercalcemia is still not a common finding even in hospital patients although its frequency may vary between 0.6% (Shek et al. 1990) and 3.6% (Keating et al. 1969).

With respect to humoral hypercalcemia of malignancy (HHM), it is often difficult or impossible to differentiate whether the patient's symptoms stem from the increased calcium levels in the blood or from the malignant disease itself which causes these increased levels (including drugs for cancer treatment) (Baechler et al. 1985). From the decrease in patient complaints after lowering the calcium levels some conclusions can be drawn retrospectively (Ralston et al. 1990).

Calcium measurements need to be performed not only in patients showing one or more of the symptoms in Table 1, but also in patients with already known neoplastic diseases when staging is done because hypercalcemia may occur without symptoms, or the symptoms may be falsely ascribed to the tumor disease. The frequency of HHM seen in the different malignancies is between less than 5% and more than 12% (Myers 1960).

Hypercalcemia is a condition which more often than expected is caused by more than one underlying disease. This is especially true for primary

Table 1. Components of the hypercalcemic syndrome

Organ	Disturbance (reversible)	Resulting symptom or complication	Destabilization to hypercalcemic crisis
Kidney	Hyposthenuria, hypercalciuria sodium, potassium loss → hypokalemia	Polyuria, polydipsia, exsiccosis, muscle weakness, arrhythmia	*Oliguria*, *anuria*, azotemia
Intestine	Increased gastric acid secretion, pancreatic enzyme secretion, delayed intestinal transport	Loss of appetite, nausea, vomiting, weight loss, constipation	(Increase)
Central nervous system	Endocrine psychic syndrome, EEG changes	Weakness, tiredness, loss of initiative, depression, dizziness, loss of appetite	*Somnolence*, *coma*
Musculature	Increase in level of neuromuscular excitability	Muscle weakness, weakened reflexes	(Increase)
Cardiovascular system	ECG: shortened QT-time	Arrhythmia (hypertension)	Cardiac arrest (avoid digitalis!)

hyperparathyroidism, which often runs for many years until it is diagnosed. If a second hypercalcemic condition then develops, the clinical manifestation of hypercalcemia may be earlier than with a single underlying disease. Therefore, primary hyperparathyroidism can be overlooked in a cancer patient in whom hypercalcemia is diagnosed as HHM (Ziegler et al. 1974; Burkhardt and Kistler 1981). The diagnostic tools of today which show decreased intact PTH in HHM and often increased PTHrP in the tumor patient lower the risk of misinterpretation. Measurable iPTH in an HHM patient is indicative of coexisting primary hyperparathyroidism.

There is no doubt that HHM develops during the later stages of a malignancy. Mostly it is a sign of poor prognosis. One decade ago 70% of HHM patients died within 1 month and more than 90% within 1 year (Burkhardt and Kistler 1981). The introduction of more efficient calcium-lowering drugs like the bisphosphonates has brought a slight improvement but no breakthrough – newer data indicate a death rate of 50% within 1 month and 75% within 3 months (Ralston et al. 1990).

Therefore, the patient's symptoms and life expectancy have to be carefully balanced. Of course it is a relief for the patient to have symptoms like nausea and vomiting removed if it is possible. On the other hand, calling back a patient with intractable cancer disease from merciful somnolence to more suffering from cancer pain may be the wrong decision. It has to be kept in mind that, among the spectrum of conditions which may cause the death of the cancer patient, hypercalcemia is regarded as one of the "least worst deaths" (Battin 1983). The obligation to minimize suffering in all patients (Boisaubin et al. 1991) may include the doctor's decision not to treat HHM in spite of the availability of potent drugs.

Kidney

The kidney is an important organ for calcium homeostasis: during hypocalcemia calcium excretion is diminished due to increased PTH, during nonparathyroid-related hypercalcemia the kidney serves as a calcium overflow, and calcium excretion may increase fivefold over normal to get rid of the calcium load (Mundy 1987). However, if hypercalcemia is caused by PTH or substances with identical biological activity like PTHrP, the hormone-induced increase in tubular calcium reabsorption in part counteracts the overflow phenomenon. Nevertheless, hypercalciuria persists and is accompanied by increased sodium and also potassium excretion – hypertonic diuresis leads to polyuria which causes polydipsia as a frequent symptom of the hypercalcemic patient ("diabetes hypercalciaemicus"). Higher grades of hypercalcemia impair the excretional capacity of the tubular apparatus leading to hyposthenuria and, later on especially when exsiccosis develops, azotemia. Interestingly, patients with HHM already show the beginnings of renal insufficiency at grades of hypercalcemia which still do not impair kidney function when caused by primary hyperparathyroidism (Burkhardt and Kistler 1981). Perhaps the vasoactive dilatative activity of PTH (Mok et al. 1989) prevents earlier kidney damage (Lins 1979). Whether PTHrP exerts the same protective effect is uncertain. Potassium loss during hypercalciuria may lead to muscle weakness and cardiac arrhythmia (see below).

In spite of more severe disturbances of kidney function compared to primary hyperparathyroidism, HHM shows a good reversibility of the impairment if plasma calcium is lowered: of the individual symptoms in a group of HHM patients, renal symptoms showed an 83% reduction after antihypercalcemic therapy (Ralston et al. 1990). This experience is of great importance for therapeutic decisions with respect to the use of drugs which require sufficient renal clearance.

Intestine

Hypercalcemia affects several gastrointestinal organs: it increases gastric acid secretion (perhaps via the stimulation of gastrin) and pancreatic enzyme and calcium excretion – however, manifestations of hypercalcemic primary hyperparathyroidism like peptic gastroduodenal ulcers or calcifying pancreatitis do not commonly accompany HHM. Perhaps the duration of hypercalcemia is too short to generate these complications (which are not too frequent even in primary hyperparathyroidism). Furthermore, hypercalcemia increases the level of neuromuscular excitability. Whereas hypocalcemia can lead to visceral tetany, spasms and accelerated stools, hypercalcemia may induce constipation. Whether the common loss of appetite of the hypercalcemic patient is the consequence of the disturbed function of the gastrointestinal tract or a more central nervous phenomenon is uncertain. The higher serum calcium level rises, the more often nausea and even vomiting may occur. Weight loss is the frequent result which not only can be seen in cancer patients in whom other factors contribute but also in patients with primary hyperparathyroidism. Clinically, the combination of symptoms such as polyuria and polydipsia together with weight loss may at first glance resemble diabetes mellitus.

When hypercalcemia was treated in HHM patients, constipation was improved in 70% of patients, nausea and vomiting in 56%, and anorexia in 50% (Ralston et al. 1990). If we presume that constipation is mainly dependent on the degree of hypercalcemia (such as kidney function, see above) and therefore more frequently improved when calcium level is lowered, the other gastrointestinal symptoms seem to be caused to a considerable extent by the tumor disease itself, and this component is not influenced by normalizing blood calcium.

Central Nervous System and Musculature

It is well known that primary hyperparathyroidism causes an endocrine psychic syndrome, depending on the degree of hypercalcemia (Herrmann et al. 1983), which is characterized by weakness and tiredness, loss of initiative, and even depression. Loss of appetite may be part of this complex. If calcium rises further, consciousness may be lost (see "Hypercalcemic Cisis" below). Nonspecific changes of the EEG may be seen – in tumor patients the question of cerebral metastases often arises (March et al. 1991). Hypercalcemia-induced symptoms promptly vanish after plasma calcium is normalized. Muscle weakness may have a central nervous origin; on the other hand hypercalcemia increases the level of neuromuscular excitation. The reflex level is high, and even areflexia may develop. A further factor contributing to diminished muscle strength is hypokalemia. Diminished muscle strength is distinctly improved after successful surgery in primary hyperparathyroidism (Kristoffersson et al. 1992). Central nervous symptoms respond quite well to anithypercalcemic treatment – an improvement can be expected in 71% of cases (Ralston et al. 1990).

Cardiovascular System

It is surprising how well the heart tolerates hypercalcemia; the heart muscle reacts to increased calcium similarly to its reaction to digitalis – this explains why, e.g., a heavy fluid load is tolerated during the diuretic treatment of hypercalcemia. On the other hand, the summative effect of hypercalcemia plus digitalis may lead to cardiac arrest. Therefore, digitalis is contraindicated (and superfluous) in patients with hypercalcemia. The ECG may show a typical shortening of the QT-time, but this sign is only present in about 20% of patients. In primary hyperparathyroidism hypertension is somewhat more frequently seen than in normocalcemics – however, there are no relevant data for HHM patients available.

Underlying Disease

Patients with HHM present with a mixture of symptoms in part due to hypercalcemia in part due to the individual malignancy (Baechler et al. 1985). Many disturbances and complaints can be caused by both conditions – this is especially true for general malaise, fatigue and weakness as well as loss of appetite and weight loss.

Hypercalcemia itself is painless – therefore, pains indicate manifestation in the organs of the underlying disease. Bone pains are indicative of skeletal metastases – however, advanced primary hyperparathyroidism also leads to bone lesions. Painful ankles may be caused by pseudogout as a symptom of primary hyperparathyroidism; in HHM it is rare. Unspecific pain may stem from paraneoplastic polyneuropathy, and it is indicative that in contrast to other symptoms pain is not relieved after successful lowering of blood calcium (Ralston et al. 1990). Whether moderate hypercalcemia increases pain threshold is unknown – the loss of consciousness is, of course, accompanied by analgesia.

Drugs

As previously mentioned, digitalis is contraindicated in HHM and may cause cardiac complications. Further disadvantagous drugs are thiazides; they diminish calcium excretion, leading to worsening hypercalcemia and its symptoms. The furosemide type is the primary line of diuretic treatment during hypercalcemia. Of the drugs which are used for the treatment of advanced breast cancer, tamoxifen deserves special attention with respect to calcium homeostasis: some women with bone metastases may develop hypercalcemia with typical symptoms after initiation of tamoxifen treatment (Villalon et al. 1979; Bezwoda et al. 1980). Symptoms due to hypercalcemia may limit the use of drugs which are useful for the condition itself as well as the underlying disease. Nausea and vomiting will prevent oral treatment of hypercalcemia with sufficient quantities of fluid or with drugs like the bisphosphonates which may cause gastrointestinal complaints – however, the availability of preparations for intravenous use solves this problem (Thiébaud et al. 1986; Scharla et al. 1987).

Hypercalcemic Crisis

Stable hypercalcemia may destabilize to a crisis if exsiccosis occurs – this may be the case when a hypercalcemic patient with polydipsia is nauseous and vomiting and cannot drink. The cardinal symptoms of hypercalcemic crisis are progressive renal insufficiency (oliguria, anuria) accompanied by somnolence and coma (see Table 1).

If a hypercalcemic crisis develops it is most frequently caused by primary hyperparathyroidism although this disease is only responsible for about 20% of cases of hypercalcemia (Burkhardt and Kistler 1981). Presumably this relationship will slowly change: primary hyperparathyroidism nowadays is diagnosed about 10 years earlier than 1 or 2 decades ago (Raue et al. 1989), and parathyrotoxic crisis is now a rare event because the supply of parenteral fluid to critically ill patients starts earlier than in the past. On the other hand, tumor patients survive longer and therefore will more often also develop hypercalcemia as an end stage complication. Thus, hypercalcemia can be regarded as a "marker of advanced cancer" although it is less frequently directly responsible for death (11 out of a group of 40 patients, Ralston et al. 1990). Again, the physician taking care of a hypercalcemic patient has to decide whether "to do everything" to lower blood calcium or whether to do "something" including fluid supply but without forcing calcium down in case the patient is already in extremis and will not profit from achieving normocalcemia for a short period (Boisaubin et al. 1991).

References

Baechler R, Sauter C, Honegger HP, Oelz O (1985) Hypercalciämie bei Non-Hodgkin-Lymphomen. Schweiz Med Wochenschr 115:332–334

Battin MB (1983) The least worst death. Hasting Center Rep 13:13–16

Bezwoda WR, Derman D, Zaltzman M, de Moor NG, Lange M (1980) Tamoxifen and hypercalcaemia. S Afr Med J 58:821–822

Boisaubin EV, Lynch GR, Dresser R (1991) Hypercalcemia of advanced malignancy: decision making and the quality of death. Am J Med Sci 301:314–318

Burkhardt E, Kistler HJ (1981) Hypercalciämie bei hospitalisierten Patienten. Schweiz Med Wochenschr 111:2017–2023

Herrmann JM, Schonecke OW, Raue F, Ziegler R (1983) Primärer Hyperparathyroidismus. Psychische Faktoren vor und nach Parathyroidektomie. Munch Med Wochenschr 125:369–371

Keating FRJ, Jones JD, Elevback LR (1969) Distribution of serum calcium and phosphorus values in unselected ambulatory patients. J Lab Clin Med 74:507–514

Kristoffersson A, Boström A, Söderberg T (1992) Muscle strength is improved after parathyroidectomy in patients with primary hyperparathyroidism. Br J Surg 79: 165–168

Lins LE (1979) Renal function in hypercalcemia. A clinical and experimental study. Acta Med Scand [Suppl] 632:1–46

March R, Ulin R, Puccio C, Savino J, Arlin Z, Ahmed T, Mittelman A (1991) Hypercalcemia associated with adenocarcinoma of the rectum. A case report and review of the literature. Anticancer Res 11:2029–2030

Mok LLS, Nickols GA, Thompson JC, Cooper CW (1989) Parathyroid hormone as a smooth muscle relaxant. Endocrine Rev 10:420–436
Mundy GR (1987) The hypercalcemia of malignancy. Kidney Int 31:142–155
Myers WPL (1960) Hypercalcemia in neoplastic disease. Arch Surg 80:308–318
Ralston SH, Gallacher SJ, Campbell J, Boyle IT (1990) Cancer-associated hypercalcemia. Morbidity and mortality. Ann Intern Med 112:499–504
Raue F, Jacubeit T, Minne H, Herfarth C, Ziegler R (1989) Primärer Hyperparathyreoidismus – Änderung eines Krankheitsbildes. Med Klin 84:178–182
Scharla SH, Minne HW, Sattar P, Mende U, Blind E, Schmidt-Gayk H, Wüster C, Ho T, Ziegler R (1987) Therapie der Tumorhypercalciämie und Clodronat. Dtsch Med Wochenschr 112:1121–1125
Shek CC, Natkunam A, Tsang V, Cockram CS, Swaminathan R (1990) Incidence, causes and mechanism of hypercalcaemia in a hospital population in Hong Kong. QJ Med 77:1277–1285
Thiébaud D, Portmann L, Jaeger P, Jacquet AF, Burckhardt P (1986) Oral versus intravenous AHPrBP (APD) in the treatment of hypercalcemia of malignancy. Bone 7:247–253
Villalon AH, Tattersall MHN, Fox RM, Woods RL (1979) Hypercalcaemia after tamoxifen for breast cancer: a sign of tumour response? Br Med J 2:1329–1330
Ziegler R, Minne H, Schultheis KH, Feyen H (1974) Das diagnostische Problem eines primären Hyperparathyreoidismus bei anderen hypercalciämischen Erkrankungen. Verh Dtsch Ges Inn Med 80:1365–1368

Hypercalcemia Associated with Hematologic Malignancies

A. Grauer

Department of Internal Medicine I – Endocrinology and Metabolism, University of Heidelberg, Bergheimerstraße 58, 69115 Heidelberg, Germany

Introduction

The estimated annual incidence rate of hypercalcemia of malignancy is about 150 new cases per million population per year (Mundy et al. 1980). It is likely to affect 20%–40% of patients with malignancies during the course of their disease. The incidence of hypercalcemia of malignancy varies between 0.07% in a population-based study of one million inhabitants (Mundy et al. 1980) and 1.1% in a large epidemiological study of hospital in- and outpatients performed at a major cancer hospital (Vassilopoulou-Sellin et al. 1993).

In this study hematologic malignancies, although not as frequent as lung, breast or gastrointestinal cancers, were characterized by a comparatively high incidence of hypercalcemia (Table 1). Hypercalcemia appears to be more frequent in multiple myeloma and in adult T-cell leukemia/lymphoma and less frequent in other hematologic conditions such as leukemia and non-Hodgkin's or Hodgkin's lymphoma. From a clinical standpoint hypercalcemia associated with malignancy has been divided into four major groups. In the first group hypercalcemia is associated with solid tumors which may or may not be accompanied with osseous metastases. This type of hypercalcemia is found in patients with lung, renal or ovarian cancer and is usually called hypercalcemia of malignancy. In the second group are solid tumors associated with extensive bone metastases, the most frequent clinical entity being breast cancer. A combination of impaired glomerular filtration and increased bone resorption is found in the disease representing the third group of hypercalcemias associated with malignancy, myeloma. The fourth group consists of lymphomas, where hypercalcemia, at least in some cases, seems to be due to increased absorption of calcium from the gut, together with increased bone resorption as in lymphomas associated with elevated 1,25-$(OH)_2D_3$ levels (Mundy 1988). Recent data suggest, however, that the different groups share the underlying mechanisms involved in the de-

Table 1. Incidence of hypercalcemia in hematologic malignancies. (Vassilopoulou-Sellin et al. 1993)

Malignancy	Patients tested	Patients with hypercalcemia		
		Total	Moderate (%) (2.7–3.0 m*M*)	Severe (%) (>3.0 m*M*)
All malignancies	7667	88 (1.15%)	48 (0.63%)	40 (0.52%)
Multiple myeloma	126	4 (3.17%)	3 (2.38%)	1 (0.79%)
Non-Hodgkin's lymphoma	381	4 (1.05%)	3 (0.79%)	1 (0.26%)
Leukemia	473	6 (1.26%)	3 (0.63%)	3 (0.63%)

velopment of hypercalcemia at least to some extent, adding even more complexity to the pathogenesis of hypercalcemia of malignancy.

Multiple Myeloma

Multiple myeloma is characterized by the neoplastic proliferation of a single clone of plasma cells engaged in the production of a monoclonal immunoglobulin. This clone of plasma cells proliferates in the bone marrow and frequently invades the adjacent bone, leading to bone pain, fractures and hypercalcemia. Approximately one-third of the patients with multiple myeloma develop hypercalcemia at some time during the course of their disease (Mundy and Martin 1982), which is always associated with extensive bone destruction occurring adjacent to myeloma cell clusters. Skeletal X-rays reveal abnormalities in 79% of patients. These consist of diffuse osteopenia, lytic lesions, and fractures, with over half of patients having a combination of all three.

The bone resorption leading to hypercalcemia in myeloma is caused by bone-resorbing cytokines secreted by myeloma cells previously circumscribed by the term "osteoclast activating factor" (Mundy et al. 1974). A number of these cytokines have now been identified and include interleukin I (IL-1), tumor necrosis factor α (TNFα, cachectin), and tumor necrosis factor β (TNFβ, lymphotoxin). Lymphotoxin appears to play a central part in this mechanism. Most, but not all of the bone-resorbing activity from several human myeloma cell lines could be selectively inhibited by antibodies to lymphotoxin, whereas there was no evidence of TNFα and IL-1 actions (Garrett et al. 1987). As not all of the bone-resorbing activity could be neutralized by lymphotoxin antibodies, it is likely that other factors are also involved. These could be produced by the myeloma cells and are yet to be identified, or they could be produced by normal immune cells in response to the presence of the malignant myeloma cells. Interleukin 6 (IL-6), a growth factor for myeloma cells, which is produced in excessive amounts in patients with severe myeloma, could be one of the possible agents, either alone or in conjunction with IL-1 or TNFα (Yoneda et al. 1993). Although essentially all patients with myeloma have extensive bone destruction, only some develop hypercalcemia. Moreover, there is no direct positive correlation between the amount of bone-resorbing activity produced by myeloma cells in vitro and the serum calcium concentration (Durie et al. 1981). An impairment of renal function is most likely a major pathogenetic feature of multiple myeloma. Proteinuria is present in almost 90% and urinary light chain (Bence-Jones) proteinuria is detected in 80% of myeloma patients. The monoclonal light chains precipitate in the distal and collecting tubules of the kidney as large, waxy, laminated casts, characteristic for the "myeloma kidney" (Kyle 1989). The impairment of the renal function – the serum cretinine value is increased initially in almost half of the patients – leads to a diminished renal clearance of calcium and promotes the development of hypercalcemia, which in turn contributes to the deterioration of renal function, leading to renal failure (Kyle 1989).

Malignant Lymphomas

Occasional patients with various lymphomas develop hypercalcemia. This occurs occasionally in Hodgkin's disease, in B-cell lymphomas, and in Burkitt's lymphoma but is fairly common among the rare subgroup of adult T-cell leukemia/lymphoma. In these diseases bone lesions are far more common than hypercalcemia, which although most often associated with bone involvement and related to direct tumor invasion of bone, can also occur in the absence of lytic lesions in bone consistent with a humoral mechanism (Martin and Grill 1992).

Hodgkin's Lymphoma

Hypercalcemia appears to be rare in this disease; when it does occur, it is most likely in patients with extensive disease with a large tumor bulk. Out of 190 consecutive patients with stage III ($n = 81$) and stage IV ($n = 109$), only one patient of these presented with hypercalcemia, despite the presence of bone lesions in 34 patients (Canellos 1974). To presume a role for vitamin D in the pathogenesis of hypercalcemia in Hodgkin's disease was prompted by the observation that intake of low doses of vitamin D led to hypercalcemia in a patient with Hodgkin's disease. After withdrawal of vitamin D hypercalcemia abated, but recurred later with the progression of the disease (Kabakow et al. 1957). Convincing evidence that $1,25\text{-}(OH)_2D_3$ was the predominant factor in the pathophysiology of this condition was provided by an observation of a patient with Hodgkin's disease whose hypercalcemia became worse on sunlight exposure in the presence of high levels of 1,25-$(OH)_2D_3$. After successful chemotherapy the patient improved and hypercalcemia disappeared. Reexposure to sunlight provoked an increase in 25-OHD_3 but not of 1,25-$(OH)_2D_3$. This led to the conclusion that lymphoma tissue may possess 1-α-hydroxylase activity (Davies et al. 1985), which has been supported by other observations (Schaefer et al. 1986; Zaloga et al. 1985).

Non-Hodgkin's Lymphoma

With the exception of the adult T-cell leukemia/lymphoma, hypercalcemia is also a rare event in non-Hodgkin's lymphoma. Due to the heterogeneity of the clinical entity, the pathogenesis, if unraveled, is variable. Again bone lesions are more frequent in these conditions than hypercalcemia. This is especially true for *Burkitt's lymphoma*, which occurs most frequently – associated with Epstein-Barr virus infections – in the jaws of African children or associated with preceding immune dysfunction, e.g., AIDS. It is almost always associated with local osteoclastic bone resorption; hypercalcemia, however, has been reported only in one single case so far (Spiegel et al. 1978). A suppression of endogenous PTH has been reported in this case, and the mechanism of hypercalcemia in these patients remains to be elucidated.

In other non-Hodgkin's lymphomas increased levels of 1,25-$(OH)_2D_3$ have been found to cause hypercalcemia (Mudde et al. 1987). In contrast to hypercalcemia in Hodgkin's disease, this occurred predominantly in the absence of detectable bone involvement (Breslau et al. 1984; Rosenthal et al. 1985). For *B-cell lymphomas*, which represent the majority of non-Hodgkin's lymphomas only few cases have been reported, where other pathogenetic factors causing hypercalcemia have been identified. PTHrP is one of these factors; elevated levels have been found in two hypercalcemic patients in a Japanese study (Nakamura et al. 1992). Coincidental mechanisms, however, such as the production of bone-resorbing cytokines by the lymphoid cells may also be involved (Mundy 1988).

Adult-T-Cell Leukemia/Lymphoma (ATLL)

In this subgroup of lymphoma patients hypercalcemia is unusually common. This disease has a predominant geographic distribution in Japan and a small cluster in the West Indies (Catovsky et al. 1982), but it also present in other parts of the world (Blayney et al. 1983). The disease is characterized by high white blood cell counts, frequent and rapidly progressive skin lesions, lymphadenopathy, and hepatosplenomegaly. It is strongly associated with a type C retrovirus, the human T-cell lymphotrophic virus type 1 (HTLV-1).

Hypercalcemia is reported in 50%–100% of these patients and appears to be the most important diagnostic prognostic determinant in this disease and a frequent cause of death. Hypercalcemia can lead to acute pancreatitis (Dazai et al. 1991) and the development of metastatic calcifications (Senba and Kawai 1991) in these patients. It occurs in the presence of elevated alkaline phosphatase levels and with an increased uptake in ^{99m}Tc-bone scans, suggestive of metabolic bonedisease with an increased bone turnover. In some patients focal bone lesions can also be identified, which appear to be due to local osteolytic activity and not to tumor infiltration (Bunn et al. 1983). There are case reports demonstrating elevated 1,25-$(OH)_2D_3$ levels in some patients with this disease (Breslau et al. 1984; Rosenthal et al. 1985). It was even possible to demonstrate the capacity of HTLV-1 transformed cord blood lymphocytes to metabolize 25-OHD_3 and produce 1,25-$(OH)_2D_3$. Recent evidence suggests, however, that 1,25-$(OH)_2D_3$ is at least not the only important pathogenetic agent causing hypercalcemia in these patients, since it has been found to be normal or even suppressed in other patients (Adams et al. 1989; Motokura et al. 1989). The demonstration of PTH-like activity and PTHrP mRNA levels in adult T-cell lymphoma cells (Motokura et al. 1989), PTHrP protein in neoplastic tissue of HTLV-1 positive ATLL (Mosely et al. 1991) and elevated serum levels of PTHrP in hypercalcemic patients with ATLL (Nakamura et al. 1992) makes it likely that PTHrP either alone or in combination with 1,25-$(OH)_2D_3$ (Johnston and Hammond 1992) or interleukin 1α (Sato et al. 1989) plays a role in the development of bone resorption and hypercalcmia in ATLL. This is supported by recent evidence that an HTLV-1 protein designated *tax* can lead to a transactivation of the PTHrP gene (Watanabe et al. 1990) and that the PTHrP gene expression in HTLV-1-infected cells is stimulated by cAMP-dependent pathways (Ikeda et al. 1993). The detection of elevated levels of TNFα (Matsuda et al. 1990) and TNFβ (Ishibashi et al. 1992) in sera of patients with ATLL demonstrate the apparent variability and/or complexity of the pathomechanism of hypercalcemia in ATLL,which will have to be further investigated.

Leukemia

With the exception of the HTLV-1-associated forms of leukemia, hypercalcemia is a rare complication of chronic and acute leukemia (Table 1) (Canellos 1974; Matsuda et al. 1990; Nakamura et al. 1992; Vassilopoulou-Sellin et al. 1993), chronic lymphatic leukemia being the most common among the uncommon causes of hypercalcemia (Hennemann et al. 1987). There are single case reports where osteoclastic bone resorption was identified in bone biopsies (Norby and Vikrot 1975). The mechanism responsible for hypercalcemia in non-HTLV-1-associated leukemias, however, is unclear. Ectopic PTH production (Cohn et al. 1987), elevated PTHrP levels

(Maruyama et al. 1992) and PGE_2 (Todo et al. 1987) appear to be possible pathogenetic principles.

References

Adams JS, Fernandez M, Gacad MA, Gill PS, Endres DB, Rasheed S, Singer FS (1989) Vitamin D metabolite-mediated hypercalcemia and hypercalciuria patients with AIDS- and non-AIDS-associated lymphoma. Blood 73:235–239

Blayney DW, Jaffe ES, Blattner WA, Cossman J, Robert GM, Longo DL, Bunn P Jr, Gallo RC (1983) The human T-cell leukemia/lymphoma virus associated with American adult T-cell leukemia/lymphoma. Blood 62:401–405

Breslau NA, McGuire JL, Zerwekh JE, Frenkel EP, Pak CY (1984) Hypercalcemia associated with increased serum calcitriol levels in three patients with lymphoma. Ann Intern Med 100:1–6

Bunn P Jr, Schechter GP, Jaffe E, Blayney D, Young RC, Matthews MJ, Blattner W, Bvoder S, Robert GM, Gallo RC (1983) Clinical course of retrovirus-associated adult T-cell lymphoma in the United States. N Engl J Med 309:257–264

Canellos GP (1974) Hypercalcemia in malignant lymphoma and leukemia. Ann NY Acad Sci 230:240–246

Catovsky D, Greaves MF, Rose M, Galton DA, Goolden AW, McCluskey DR, White JM, Lampert I, Bourikas G, Ireland R, Brownell AI, Bridges JM, Blattner WA, Gallo RC (1982) Adult T-cell lymphoma-leukaemia in Blacks from the West Indies. Lancet 1:639–643

Cohn SL, Morgan ER, Mallette LE (1987) The spectrum of metabolic bone disease in lymphoblastic leukemia. Cancer 59:346–350

Davies M, Mawer EB, Hayes ME, Lumb GA (1985) Abnormal vitamin D metabolism in Hodgkin's lymphoma. Lancet 1:1186–1188

Dazai Y, Katoh I, Hara Y, Yoshida R, Kurihara K (1991) Two cases of adult T-cell leukemia associated with acute pancreatitis due to hypercalcemia. Am J Med 90:251–254

Durie BGM, Salmon SE, Mundy GR (1981) Relation of osteoclast activating factor production to the extent of bone disease in multiple myeloma. Br J Haematol 47:21–30

Garrett IR, Durie BG, Nedwin GE, Gillespie A, Bringman T, Sabatini M, Bertolini DR, Mundy GR (1987) Production of lymphotoxin, a bone-resorbing cytokine, by cultured human myeloma cells. N Engl J Med 317:526–532

Hennemann HH, Hastka J, Lengfelder E, Pfiester P, Bonatz K (1987) Hypercalcemias in chronic lymphatic leukemias and other non-Hodgkin's lymphomas. Klin Wochenschr 65:791–797

Ikeda K, Okazaki R, Inoue D, Ogata E, Matsumoto T (1993) Transcription of the gene for parathyroid hormone-related peptide from the human is activated through a cAMP-dependent pathway by prostaglandin E1 in HTLV-I-infected T cells. J Biol Chem 268:1174–1179

Ishibashi K, Kodama M, Hanada S, Arima T (1992) Tumor necrosis factor beta and hypercalcemia. Leuk Lymphoma 7:409–417

Johnston SR, Hammond PJ (1992) Elevated serum parathyroid hormone related protein and 1,25-dihydroxycholecalciferol in hypercalcaemia associated with adult T-cell leukaemia-lymphoma. Postgrad Med J 68:753–755

Kabakow B, Mines MF, King FH (1957) Hypercalcemia in Hodgkin's disease. N Engl J Med 256:59–62

Kyle RA (1989) Monoclonal gammopathies and the kidney. Annu Rev Med 40:53–60

Martin TJ, Grill V (1992) Hypercalcemia in cancer. J Steroid Biochem Mol Biol 43:123–129
Maruyama H, Kawano K, Uno H, Matsuoka H, Yamashita R, Tamaki N, Ishizaki J, Maeda K, Tsuda K (1992) Acute lymphocytic leukemia (L1) preceded by hypercalcemia. Rinsho Ketsueki 33:514–519
Matsuda K, Yamamoto N, Kaneko N, Iwashi M, Hashimoto S, Araki K (1990) Hypercalcemia and adult T-cell leukemia (letter). Lancet 335:1032
Mosely JM, Danks JA, Grill V, Lister TA, Horton MA (1991) Immunocytochemical demonstration of PTHrP protein in neoplastic tissue of HTLV-1 positive human adult T-cell leukemia/lymphoma: implications for the mechanism of hypercalcemia. Br J Cancer 64:745–748
Motokura T, Fukumoto S, Matsumoto T, Takahashi S, Fujita A, Yamashita T, Igarashi T, Ogata E (1989) Parathyroid hormone-related protein in adult T-cell leukemia-lymphoma. Ann Intern Med 111:484–488
Mudde AH, van den Berg H, Boshuis PG, Breedveld FC, Markusse HM, Kluin PM, Bijvoet OL, Papapoulos SE (1987) Ectopic production of 1,25-dihydroxyvitamin D by B-cell lymphoma as a cause of hypercalcemia. Cancer 59:1543–1546
Mundy GR (1988) Hypercalcemia of malignancy revisited. J Clin Invest 82:1–6
Mundy GR, Martin TJ (1982) The hypercalcemia of malignancy: pathogenesis and management. Metabolism 31:1247–1277
Mundy GR, Raisz LG, Cooper RA, Schlechter GP, Salmon SE (1974) Evidence for the secretion of an osteoclast stimulating factor in myeloma. N Engl J Med 291:1041–1046
Mundy GR, Cove DH, Fisken R (1980) Primary hyperparathyroidism: changes in the pattern of clinical presentation. Lancet 1:1317–1320
Nakamura Y, Bando H, Shintani Y, Yokogoshi Y, Saito S (1992) Serum parathyroid hormone-related protein concentrations in patients with hematologic malignancies or solid tumors. Acta Endocrinol (Copenh) 127:324–330
Norby K, Vikrot O (1975) Hypercalcemia in chronic lymphatic leukemia. Scand J Haematol 15:132–138
Rosenthal N, Insogna KL, Godsall JW, Smaldone L, Waldron JA, Stewart AF (1985) Elevations in circulating 1,25-dihydroxyvitamin D in three patients with lymphoma-associated hypercalcemia. J Clin Endocrinol Metab 60:29–33
Sato K, Fujii Y, Kasono K, Ozawa M, Imamura H, Kanaji Y, Kuroxawa H, Tsushima T, Shizume K (1989) Parathyroid hormone related protein and interleukin 1-alpha synergistically stimulate bone resorption in vitro and increase the serum calcium concentration in vivo. Endocrinology 124:2172–2178
Schaefer K, Saupe J, Pauls A, von Herrath D (1986) Hypercalcemia and elevated serum 1,25-dihydroxyvitamin D_3 in a patient with Hodgkin's lymphoma. Klin Wochenschr 64:89–91
Senba M, Kawai K (1991) Metastatic calcification due to hypercalcemia in adult T-cell leukemia-lymphoma (ATLL). Zentralbl Pathol 137:341–345
Spiegel A, Greene M, Magrath I, Balow J, Marx S, Auerbach GD (1978) Hypercalcemia with suppressed parathyroid hormone in Burkitt's lymphoma. Am J Med 64:691–702
Todo S, Imashuku S, Inoda H, Yamanaka H, Hibi S, Tsunamoto K, Esumi N, Fujiwara F, Shimizu Y, Morioka Y (1987) Hypercalcemia in a case of childhood acute lymphoblastic leukemia. Jpn J Clin Oncol 17:357–362
Vassilopoulou-Sellin R, Newman BM, Taylor SH, Guinee VF (1993) Incidence of hpercalcemia in patients with malignancy referred to a comprehensive cancer center. Cancer 71:1309–1312
Watanabe T, Yamaguchi K, Takatsuki K, Osame M, Yoshida M (1990) Constitutive expression of parathyroid hormone-related protein gene in human T cell leukemia

virus type 1 (HTLV-1) carriers and adult T cell leukemia patients that can be transactivated by HTLV-1 tax gene. J Exp Med 172:759–765
Yoneda T, Nakai M, Moriyama K, Scott L, Ida N, Kunitomo T, Mundy GR (1993) Neutralizing antibodies to human interleukin 6 reverse hypercalcemia associated with a human squamous carcinoma. Cancer Res 53:737–740
Zaloga GP, Eil C, Medberry CA (1985) Humoral hypercalcemia in Hodgkin's disease: association with elevated 1,25-dihydroxycholecalciferol levels and subperiosteal bone resorption. Arch Intern Med 145:155–157

Differential Diagnosis of Hypercalcemia: Laboratory Assessment

H. Schmidt-Gayk and Heike Haerdt

Laboratory Group, Im Breitspiel 15, 69126 Heidelberg, Germany

The differential diagnosis of hypercalcemia can be very simple in many cases as well as extremely complicated and difficult in others. Initially, the history of the patient is very important as well as a physical examination and X-rays, as described by Ziegler in this volume. The laboratory assessment is based on the routine serum and urine chemistry tests.

Serum Calcium

Initially it should be ascertained whether true hypercalcemia exists; thereafter the etiology of an elevated serum calcium level has to be established. A number of biologic and analytical factors, in addition to the technique of blood collection, are known to influence the concentration of serum calcium. As about half of the serum calcium is protein bound, the existence of artifactual hypercalcemia or normocalcemia should be taken into account. Hyper- or hypoproteinemia should be ruled out (Schmidt-Gayk et al. 1991). If serum calcium is elevated and serum total protein or total protein and albumin are normal, true hypercalcemia may be assumed. We tested different formulas for the calculation of calcium corrected for protein in 214 patients with primary hyperparathyroidism (pHPT), and the results are shown in Fig. 1. Formulas for the calculation are given in the appendix.

As shown in Fig. 1, hypercalcemia in patients with pHPT was separated from the normal range (2.25–2.60 mmol/l) slightly better by correction of calcium for total protein (Husdan et al. 1973). We found no advantage in correcting the calcium for albumin (Payne et al. 1979). In our patients, as shown in Fig. 1, no normocalcemic pHPT was observed.

As many hospitals and physicians perform a screening of serum calcium in all patients, a 1%–2% incidence of hypercalcemia is observed. In addition to pathologic states as shown in Table 1, hypercalcemia may be

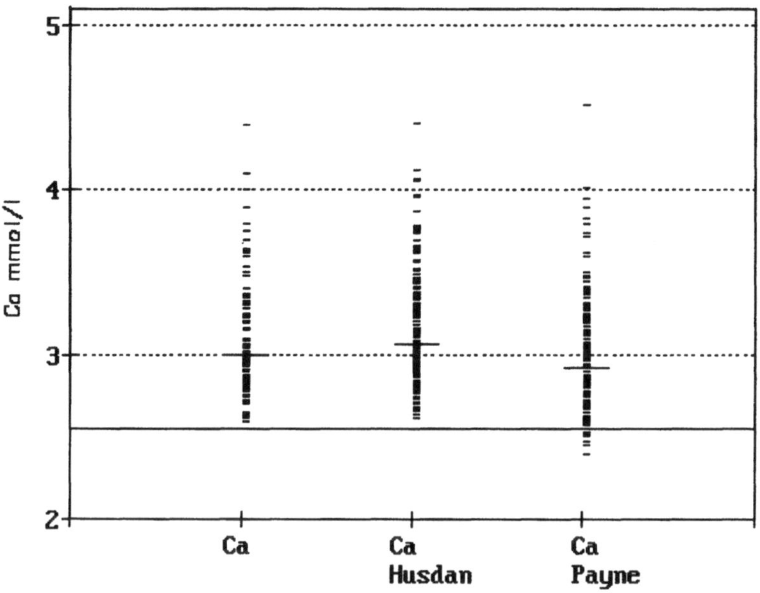

Fig. 1. Comparison of serum calcium, calcium corrected for total protein (according to Husdan et al. 1973) and calcium corrected for albumin (according to Payne et al. 1979) in 214 patients with primary hyperparathyroidism. Solid line at 2.6 mmol/l shows upper limit of normal. The median is indicated in each group

caused by laboratory error or hemoconcentration secondary to prolonged pressure of the tourniquet for venipuncture.

Ionized Plasma Calcium

Tests for the determination of ionized calcium are available for use in some hospitals. We compared three different methods for the determination of calcium in healthy controls: ionized calcium by ion selective electrode (ICA, Radiometer Copenhagen), calcium by photometry (instrument from Hitachi 717, reagents from Boehringer Mannheim, Mannheim, Germany) and total calcium by flame emission spectrophotometry (AFM, Eppendorf Geraetebau, Hamburg). Blood was taken from healthy controls at 9 a.m., 1 g calcium (Calcium Sandoz fortissimum) was given orally and serum calcium was monitored every 15 min. A statistically significant increase in serum calcium was detected earlier by flame emission spectrophotometry than by ion selective electrode or the photometric method.

Severity of hypercalcemia is of importance to the differential diagnosis. We investigated the severity of hypercalcemia in 387 patients with pHPT, 34 patients with malignancy-associated hypercalcemia (MAH), 27 patients with tertiary hyperparathyroidism (tHPT, patients on dialysis therapy with hyperparathyroidism and hypercalcemia), 8 patients on thiazide, 6 patients with vitamin D intoxication, 9 patients with multiple myeloma, and 14 patients with persistent HPT (patients after kidney transplantation with persistent HPT). The results are shown in Fig. 2, which shows the most severe hypercalcemia occurs in pHPT and in MAH. Only slight degrees of hypercalcemia (below 3.0 mmol/l) were observed in a patient with Addison's disease, a family with familial hypocalciuric hypercalcemia (FHH) (not shown in Fig. 2) and 8 patients on thiazides. Our collection of patients with multiple myeloma may be atypical, as in many cases life-threatening hypercalcemia occurs in these patients.

Chloride/Phosphate Ratio

As recommended by Palmer et al. (1974) and Reeves et al. (1975), the chloride/phosphate ratio may be used for the differential diagnosis of hypercalcemia. In patients with pHPT, chloride (normal range 96–105 mmol/l)

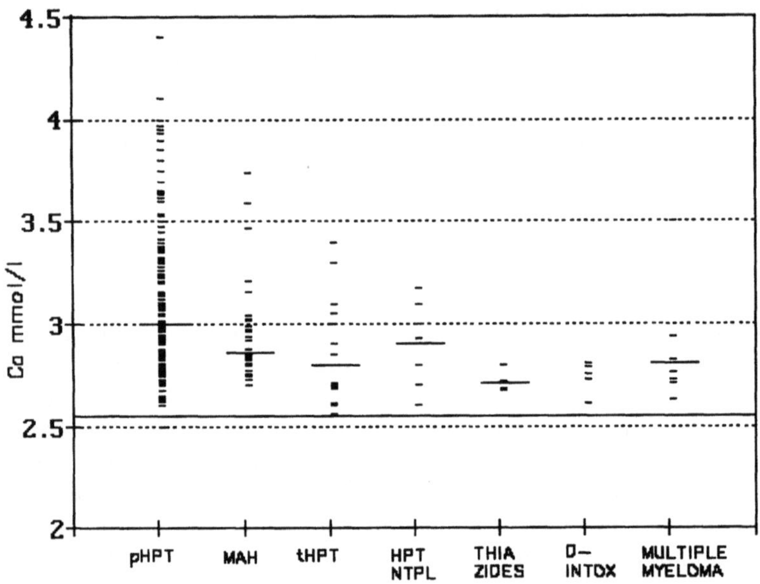

Fig. 2. Severity of hypercalcemia in different diseases showing 387 patients with primary hyperparathyroidism (*–pHPT*,median 3.0 mmol/l), 34 with malignancy-associated hypercalcemia (*MAH*, median 2.86 mmol/l), 27 with tertiary hyperparathyroidism (*tHPT*, median 2.8 mmol/l), 14 with persistent hyperparathyroidism after kidney transplantation (*HPT NTPL*, median 2.9 mmol/l), 8 patients on thiazides (median, 2.71 mmol/l), 6 with vitamin D intoxication (median, 2.75 mmol/l) and 9 with multiple myeloma (median, 2.81 mmol/l)

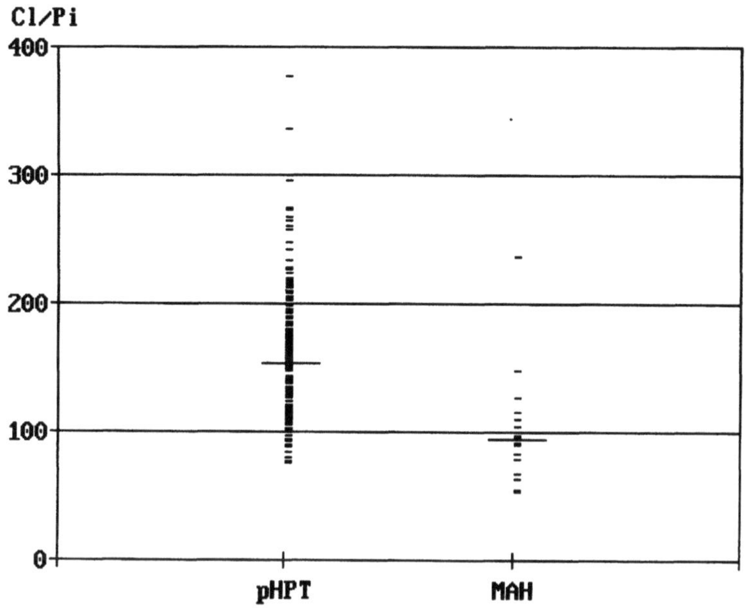

Fig. 3. Chloride/phosphate (*Cl/Pi*) ratio in 288 patients with primary hyperparathyroidism (*pHPT*) and 19 patients with malignancy-associated hypercalcemia (*MAH*)

tends to increase and phosphorus (normal range 0.8–1.5 mmol/l) tends to decrease, yielding ratios above 100, whereas in MAH the parameters may tend to go in the opposite direction. The chloride/phosphate ratio was available in 288 patients with pHPT and 19 patients with MAH; the results are shown in Fig. 3, from which it can be seen there is a considerable overlap in the chloride/phosphate ratio. In untreated patients the separation between patient groups by Cl/Pi may be slightly better; therefore this ratio may still be useful.

Phosphate

High phosphate levels are found in patients with hypercalcemia and increased intestinal phosphorus absorption, e.g., in vitamin D intoxication, sarcoidosis, and milk-alkali syndrome. High phosphate levels may also be caused by increased bone resorption, as in patients with bone metastases or in vitamin A intoxication or in tHPT patients on dialysis therapy. In tHPT, phosphorus is also elevated by decreased or zero renal phosphorus elimination.

Table 1 describes the differential diagnosis of hypercalcemia and the pathophysiology causing elevated serum calcium levels.

Table 1. Differential diagnosis and etiology of hypercalcemia. (Modified according to Shane 1993)

	Bone	Intestine	Kidney
Most common			
– HPT group			
Primary hyperparathyroidism (pHPT)	Res	Abs	Reabs
Tertiary HPT in dialysis patients	Res		
Persistent HPT after kidney TPL	Res	Abs	Reabs
Malignant disease			
– PTHrP (carcinoma of lung, renal cell, breast, esophagus, head and neck, ovary, bladder, endocrine tumors)	Res		
– Lytic bone metastases (breast carcinoma, multiple myeloma)	Res		
– Ectopic production of calcitriol (lymphoma)		Abs	
– Other factors produced locally or ectopically	Res		
Less common			
– Thyrotoxicosis	Res		
– Addison's disease			Reabs
– Granulomatous diseases		Abs	
Sarcoidosis, tuberculosis, histoplasmosis, leprosy, others			
– Drug induced			
Vitamin D		Abs	
Thiazides (common)			Reabs
Lithium	Res	Abs	Reabs
Theophylline	?		
Vitamin A	Res		
Aluminum intoxication	Ca^{2+} deposition inhibited		
Milk-alkali syndrome	Increased calcium intake		
– Immobilization	Res		
– Renal failure with rhabdomyolysis	?		
– Familial hypocalcuric hypercalcemia			Reabs

Res, increased bone resorption; Abs, increased intestinal absorption; Reabs, increased tubular reabsorption; TPL, transplant

Parathyroid Hormone

The determination of parathyroid hormone (PTH) is of the utmost importance to the differential diagnosis of hypercalcemia. For the assay of PTH, intact PTH in most laboratories has replaced the assays of the mid-regional (amino acids 44–68, Blind et al. 1988) or carboxy-terminal fragments (amino acids 53–84, Segre 1990; Schmidt-Gayk et al. 1991; Solal et al. 1991). Only rarely were the elderly amino-terminal fragment assays, mostly PTH (1–34), useful in the differential diagnosis of hypercalcemia.

The measurement of intact PTH is very reliable; however, pitfalls exist and should be taken into account (Blind et al. 1987, 1990, 1992; Nussbaum et al. 1987):

- Circadian rhythm (higher values in the evening, Herfarth et al. 1992)
- Pulsatility (a slight pulsatility is found, as published by Herfarth et al. 1992) with pulses up to 1 pmol/l in healthy persons; Harms et al. (1989) observed larger pulses.
- Increase after physical exercise (Ljunghall et al. 1988)
- Inhibition of many assays by elevated EDTA concentration (intact PTH is more stable in EDTA plasma than in serum; therefore most test kit producers recommend drawing blood into EDTA-containing tubes). If the tube is not filled with blood to the specified volume, an increased EDTA concentration is obtained causing an acid pH in the plasma. This prevents binding of the antigen to the antibody in the immunoassay and falsely low values are obtained.
- Autoantibodies (very rare; Wilkinson et al. 1990; McElduff et al. 1992)
- Human anti-mouse antibodies (HAMA, these are now occurring increasingly as patients receive monoclonal mouse antibodies in immunoscintigraphy). In most hypercalcemic patients, the two-site assay of intact PTH separates pHPT from other causes, because hypercalcemia not related to HPT suppresses PTH and values below the normal range are found (Nussbaum et al. 1987; Blind et al. 1988). Our results with intact PTH, determined with a two-site immunoradiometric assay (Blind et al. 1987) in 161 patients with surgically confirmed cases of primary hyperparathyroidism, 40 healthy controls and 27 cases of malignancy-associated hypercalcemia are shown in Fig. 4.

In about 2%–10% of the patients with surgically and histologically proven pHPT, the assay of intact PTH yields normal values, even in different samples (Nussbaum et al. 1987; Segre 1990; Ahren 1993). In rare cases, even low normal values of intact PTH were observed in pHPT (Hollenberg and Arnold 1991). These values have been determined by well-established two-site immunoassays. The question remains as to whether some patients with pHPT secrete predominantly biologically active fragments of the hormone, e.g., PTH (1–38) or similar structures (Fuleihan et al. 1989; Klee et al. 1992).

We observed a patient with histologically proven pHPT, repeatedly normal intact PTH, determined with the AllegroTM test kit (Nichols Institute, San Juan Capistrano, CA, USA), and with an assay for intact PTH similar to that used by Blind et al. 1987. This patient showed an increased level of PTH (1–38) in a newly developed two-site immunoluminometric assay (Gao and Schmidt-Gayk, in preparation). In these pHPT patients with normal intact PTH, an EDTA infusion test (Ahren and Bergenfelz 1993) or a calcium suppression test (Thome et al. 1990) may be helpful.

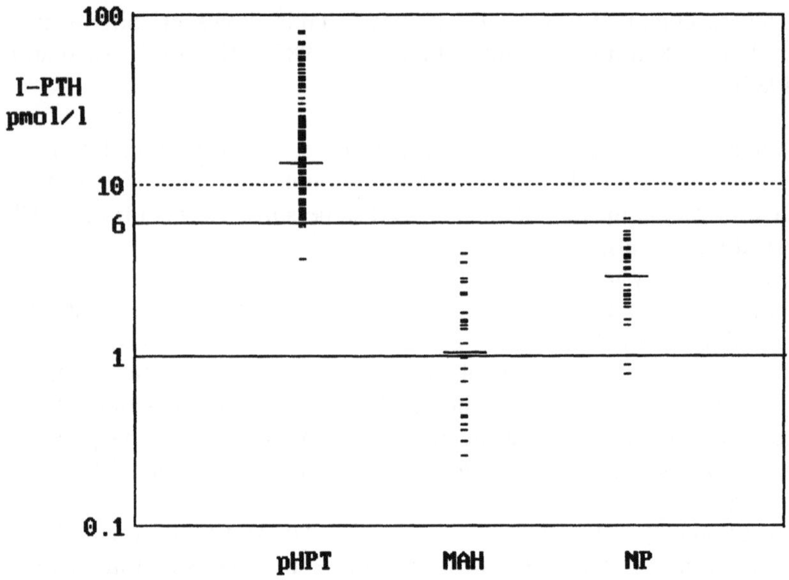

Fig. 4. Intact parathyroid hormone (*I-PTH*) in 161 patients with primary hyperparathyroidism (*pHPT*, median 13.6 pmol/l), 27 patients with malignancy-associated hypercalcemia (*MAH*, median 1.05 pmol/l) and 40 normal persons (*NP*, median 2.9 pmol/l)

In the great majority of patients hypercalcemia and elevated intact PTH are caused by pHPT. However, the following may also be responsible for elevated calcium levels and intact PTH:

- tHPT (Vosik et al. 1972)
- Persistent HPT after kidney transplantation (David et al. 1973; Bonnin et al. 1988)
- Multiple endocrine neoplasia (MEN, Marx et al. 1991)
- Familial HPT (Szabo 1993)
- Familial parathyroid carcinoma (Streeten et al. 1992)
- Ectopic PTH production by a malignant tumor (Yoshimoto et al. 1989)
- FHH (Marx et al. 1980, 1982)
- Thiazides (Krause et al. 1989)
- Lithium treatment (Birnbaum et al. 1988; Mallette et al. 1989).

Very rarely, intact PTH is produced by a tumor. We observed a case with life-threatening hypercalcemia and extremely high levels of intact PTH caused by a bronchial carcinoid. After resection of the tumor, hypercalcemia and intact PTH normalized for some time. Hypercalcemia in association with acute renal failure and rhabdomyolysis is diagnosed by history and serum calcium determination. Some cases present with serum calcium up to 4.0 mmol/l (Meneghini et al. 1993).

FHH

As hypercalcemia and elevated intact PTH occur in FHH, urinary calcium and creatinine levels have to be determined in all patients with suspected pHPT. The diagnosis of FHH may be missed if urinary calcium is not determined! Urinary creatinine level should be determined to monitor the completeness of the collection. About 20 mg creatinine is excreted per kg body wt. In addition, urinary sodium should be determined as it increases urinary calcium excretion (Shaw et al. 1992). FHH should also be excluded in cases with a history of long-lasting hypercalcemia and unsuccessful operated pHPT. This disorder is benign and most of the patients have normal intact PTH and urinary cyclic AMP. In some patients, increased intact PTH was reported. Very important for the diagnosis of FHH is the reduced excretion of calcium and magnesium, calculated best as reduced fractional renal clearance.

Serum magnesium is often elevated in this disorder. The calcium/creatinine clearance ratio is below 0.01 in most cases of FHH, whereas in pHPT this ratio exceeds 0.01 in most cases (Marx et al. 1982). Serum calcium in FHH is most often below 3.0 mmol/l; only in a few cases have levels up to 3.5 mmol/l been reported.

If the differential diagnosis is not clear at this point, X-rays of the hand should be made and subperiosteal resorption looked for, which is specific for the effect of PTH. This step should be taken initially in patients with very severe hypercalcemia, e.g., serum calcium above 4.0 mmol/l. If serum calcium is above 4.0 mmol/l and subperiosteal resorption is found, pHPT is the most probable diagnosis and the patient should be prepared for operation. For these extreme hypercalcemic cases an intact PTH assay with shortened incubation times (1–2 h) may be helpful in the differential diagnosis, if the X-rays are inconclusive.

In the case of hypercalcemia and low intact PTH, MAH should be suspected. Most often, MAH occurs during the course of the disease and the diagnosis is known. However, the diagnosis and treatment of the hypercalcemia are very important, as unrecognized hypercalcemia may be life-threatening. In a few cases hypercalcemia is the first manifestation of the tumor. If a malignancy is suspected, serum protein electrophoresis and determination of Bence-Jones protein in urine should be performed. However, there are some reports in the literature that patients with malignancy have concomitant pHPT (Farr et al. 1973; Gallacher et al. 1993). This is also the case in multiple myeloma (monoclonal gammopathy, Dexter et al. 1972). Bone marrow aspiration may be necessary in patients with suspected malignancy. If the diagnosis is unclear, a history of long duration is more indicative of pHPT than MAH. In the patient described above with pHPT presenting with normal intact PTH and elevated PTH (1–38), hypercalcemia persisted for about 3 years.

Parathyroid Hormone-Related Protein (PTHrP)

Metastatic bone disease causes hypercalcemia in many tumor patients; however, in a substantial number of patients, no metastases are found and the hypercalcemia is caused by local or systemic factors increasing bone resorption. One of the main causes of humoral hypercalcemia of malignancy is PTHrP, as described in this volume by E. Blind.

As for intact PTH, blood for PTHrP should be drawn in EDTA-containing vials for better stability. The Nichols Institute recommends the use of, and supplies, vials also containing protease inhibitors (Pandian et al. 1992). In patients with MAH an elevated PTHrP level predicts that this patient will respond less favorably to bisphosphonate treatment (Gallacher et al. 1992). A radioimmunoassay (RIA) for PTHrP (53–84) and an immunoradiometric assay (IRMA) for PTHrP (1–86) were compared by Blind et al. (1993); whereas the IRMA is much more sensitive, the number of elevated levels in patients with malignancies and hypercalcemia was higher with the RIA. A disadvantage of the RIA procedure is the dependence of this fragment on renal function (Burtis et al. 1990).

Urinary Cyclic AMP

In patients with MAH, in addition to PTHrP the determination of urinary cyclic AMP may clarify the mechanism of the hypercalcemia. In addition to PTH and PTHrP, a third factor stimulating the adenylate cyclase in the kidney might be responsible for the hypercalcemia (Fraser et al. 1993). Urinary cyclic AMP should always be determined together with creatinine clearance, as urinary cyclic AMP excretion depends on kidney function (Schmidt-Gayk et al. 1977).

Measurement of the Vitamin D Metabolites 25-Hydroxyvitamin D (25-OHD) and 1,25-Dihydroxyvitamin D (1,25-$(OH)_2$D, Calcitriol)

25-Hydroxyvitamin D

25-Hydroxyvitamin D is determined to estimate the supply of the patient with vitamin D, and largely increased levels are found in patients with vitamin D intoxication. In the widely used competitive protein-binding assays, both 25-hydroxyvitamin D_2 and 25-hydroxyvitamin D_3 are effective in displacing radiolabeled 25-OHD from the binding protein; therefore both vitamin D_2 intoxication and vitamin D_3 intoxication yield high levels of 25-OHD. The assay does not measure 1α-OHD_3, calcitriol, dihydrotachysterol (AT 10), 25-hydroxydihydrotachysterol or 5,6-*trans*-25-hydroxyvitamin D.

Calcitriol

In sarcoidosis or other granulomatous diseases, the biologically active vitamin D metabolite (calcitriol) is produced in granulomatous tissue and this production is influenced by the substrate availability, which is the amount of 25-OHD. Therefore, patients with sarcoidosis tend to be hypercalcemic only during the summer months. Angiotensin-converting enzyme activity is often elevated in patients with sarcoidosis; however, this is not a very sensitive or specific parameter.

In pHPT, the level of calcitriol in plasma also depends on the availability of 25-OHD (LoCascio et al. 1985). PTH and low phosphate levels stimulate the renal 1α-hydroxylase. As in sarcoidosis, patients with pHPT may also show increased serum calcium and calcitriol levels during the summer months or after vitamin D substitution. In contrast, PTHrP does not regulate calcitriol levels in MAH (Schilling et al. 1993). As the renal 24-hydroxylase is stimulated by hypercalcemia, patients with elevated serum calcium levels tend to have low levels of circulating 25-OHD, which are often found in patients with pHPT, as the 24-hydroxylase and the 1-hydroxylase are stimulated, resulting in increased 25-OHD consumption in this disorder (Coen et al. 1989).

In some patients with lymphoma and hypercalcemia, calcitriol is responsible for the hypercalcemia and increased serum levels have been reported in this disease (Rosenthal et al. 1985). Endogenous or exogenous calcitriol intoxication presents with hypercalcemia and hyperphosphatemia caused by increased intestinal absorption (low serum phosphate in pHPT).

Exogenous Vitamin D Intoxication

Hypercalcemia after intake of supraphysiological amounts of vitamin D depends on the concentration of free vitamin D metabolites, the activity of the 1α-hydroxylase and the degradation of vitamin D metabolites (Vieth 1990). 25-OHD in plasma is largely elevated; however, calcitriol is not consistently increased (Jacobus et al. 1992), as hyperphosphatemia and reduced kidney function decrease the activity of the 1α-hydroxylase. Hyperreactivity to vitamin D may also cause hypercalcemia. Hyperreactivity to vitamin D is also known as "idiopathic" hypercalcemia of infancy and may occur if milk is fortified with supraphysiological amounts of vitamin D

(Seelig 1970; Jacobus et al. 1992). In children, the levels of calcitriol in plasma depend to a certain extent on the substrate (25-OHD) availability. In contrast, healthy adults exhibit fairly constant plasma levels of calcitriol despite marked seasonal variation of 25-OHD. In hypoparathyroidism treated with milligram doses of vitamin D, hypercalcemia may be observed, if serum calcium is not monitored regularly or if the doses of vitamin D are increased too rapidly (Paterson 1980).

Hyperthyroidism

Thyroid hormones and TSH may be determined if hyperthyroidism is suspected as a cause of hypercalcemia. Low TSH and elevated thyroxine and triiodothyronine levels are typically found. Serum calcium concentration is usually below 3.0 mmol/l and PTH is suppressed, resulting in hyperphosphatemia (Burman et al. 1976; Bouillon and De Moor 1974).

Addison's Disease

The diagnosis of Addison's disease is made by the clinical picture and measurement of serum cortisol and ACTH. Serum calcium concentration is usually below 3.0 mmol/l. Urinary calcium concentration is low in this condition, as in FHH or patients on thiazides.

Thiazides

Preexisting hypercalcemia is exacerbated in patients with pHPT, and often hypercalcemia from 2.6 to 2.8 mmol/l is observed in other patients taking thiazides. Hypocalciuria is observed regularly (Parfitt 1969). Serum phosphate level increases slightly; however, this is not statistically significant; intact PTH rises slightly and calcitriol drops by about 30%–40% (Krause et al. 1989).

Unsolved Cases

If there are still difficulties in the differential diagnosis, the test according to Dent is of some help: 3 × 50 mg cortisone or its equivalent in glucocorticoids are given daily for 1 week and serum calcium is determined daily. Disorders with increased calcitriol formation in most cases respond rapidly and serum calcium is reversed towards normal. In addition, some patients with malignancy respond with a normalization of serum calcium, and hypercalcemia as

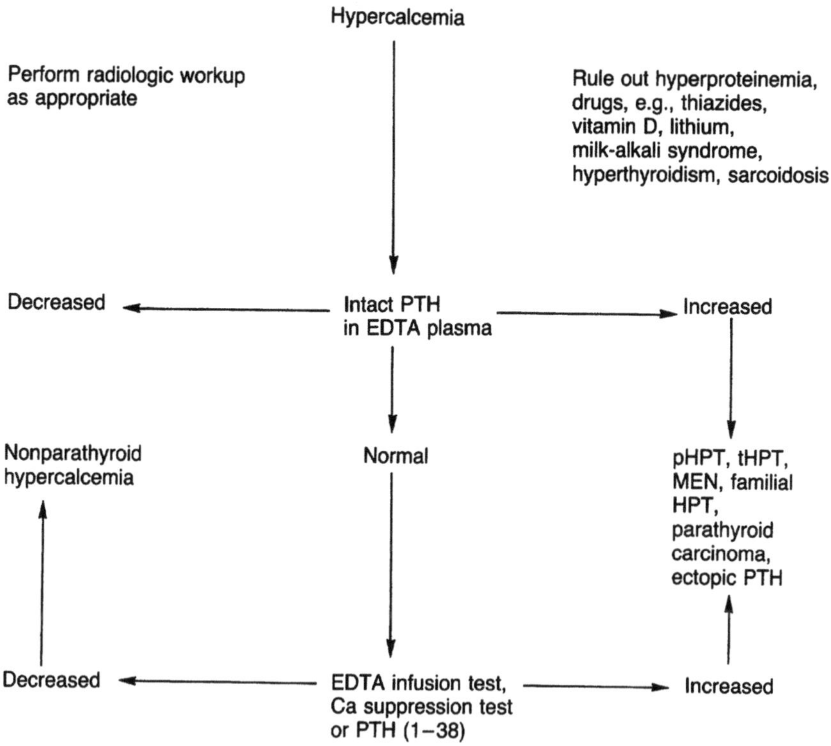

Fig. 5. Flowsheet of diagnostic workup in hypercalcemia

a consequence of Addison's disease is normalized. pHPT will not usually respond to glucocorticoids.

A stepwise procedure for the evaluation of hypercalcemia is shown in Fig. 5.

Appendix

Formulas used for the correction of total serum calcium:

1. Correction for total protein (slightly modified from Husdan et al. 1973):

$$\text{Corrected serum Ca} = \frac{\text{Measured serum calcium}}{0.6 + \dfrac{\text{Total protein (g/l)}}{194}}$$

The formula may be used for serum calcium concentration in millimoles per liter as well as for serum calcium concentration in milligrams/100 ml. If total protein is expressed in g/100 ml, it has to be divided by 19.4 (original formula from Husdan et al. 1973).

2. Correction for serum albumin (formula according to Payne et al. 1979):

Adjusted serum Ca(mmol/l) = Ca(mmol/l) − 0.025 albumin(g/l) + 1.0

or

Adjusted serum Ca(mg/100 ml) = Ca(mg/100 ml) − albumin(g/100 ml) + 4.0

References

Ahrén B, Bergenfelz A (1993) Potential clinical use of the EDTA-infusion test. Eur J Clin Chem Clin Biochem 31:353–358

Birnbaum J, Klandorf H, Giuliano A, van Herle A (1988) Lithium stimulates the release of human parathyroid hormone in vitro. J Clin Endocrinol Metab 66: 1187–1191

Blind E, Schmidt-Gayk H, Armbruster FP, Stadler A (1987) Measurement of intact human parathyrin by an extracting two-site immunoradiometric assay. Clin Chem 33:1376–1381

Blind E, Schmidt-Gayk H, Scharla S, Flentje D, Fischer S, Ghring U, Hitzler W (1988) Two-site assay of intact parathyroid hormone in the investigation of primary hyperparathyroidism and other disorders of calcium metabolism compared with a midregion assay. J Clin Endocrinol Metab 67:353–360

Blind E, Flentje D, Fischer S (1990) Clinical application of intact parathyroid hormone determination. In: Schmidt-Gayk H, Armbruster FP, Bouillon R (eds) Calcium regulating hormones, vitamin D metabolites, and cyclic Amp, assays and their clinical application. Springer, Berlin Heidelberg New York, pp 3–23

Blind E, Raue F, Reichel H (1992) Validity of intact plasma parathyrin measurements in chronic renal failure as determined by two-site immunoradiometric assays with N- or C-terminal capture antibodies. Clin Chem 38:2345–2347

Blind E, Raue F, Meinel T, Bucher M, Manegold C, Ebert W, Vogt-Moykopf I, Ziegler R (1993) Levels of parathyroid hormone-related protein in hypercalcemia of malignancy: comparison of midregional radioimmunoassay and two-site immunoradiometric assay. Clin Invest 71:31–36

Bonnin MR, Gonzalez MT, Arranz B, Rosel P, Navarro MA (1988) Intact parathyrin in patients after kidney transplantation. Clin Chem 34:2378

Bouillon R, De Moor P (1974) Parathyroid function in patients with hyper- or hypothyroidism. J Clin Endocrinol Metab 38:999–1004

Burman KD, Monchik JM, Earll JM, Wartofsky L (1976) Ionized and total serum calcium and parathyroid hormone in hyperthyroidism. Ann Intern Med 84: 668–671

Burtis WJ, Brady TG, Orlof JJ, Ersbak JB, Warrell RP, Olson BR, Wu TL, Mitnick ME, Broadus AE, Stewart AF (1990) Immunochemical characterization of circulating parathyroid hormone-related protein in patients with humoral hypercalcemia of cancer. N Engl J Med 322:1106–1112

Coen G, Bondatti F, de Matteis A, Ballanti P, Mazzaferro S, Sardella D, Smacchi A (1989) Severe vitamin D deficiency in a case of primary hyperparathyroidism caused by parathyroid lipoadenoma, effect of $25OHD_3$ treatment. Miner Electrolyte Metab 15:332–337

David DS, Sakai S, Brennan L, Riggio RA, Cheigh J, Stenzel KH, Rubin AL, Sherwood LM (1973) Hypercalcemia after renal transplantation, long-term follow-up data. N Engl Med 289:398–401

Dexter RN, Mullinax F, Estep HL, Williams RC (1972) Monoclonal IgG gammopathy and hyperparathyroidism. Ann Intern Med 77:759–764
Farr HW, Fahey TJ, Nash AG, Farr CM (1973) Primary hyperparathyroidism and cancer. Am J Surg 126:539–543
Fraser WD, Firek Ahren, Robinson Z, Lawton R, Durham B, Gallacher SZ, Boyle IT, Beastall GH, Logue FC (1993) Clinical and laboratory studies of a new immunoradiometric assay of parathyroid hormone-related protein. Clin Chem 39:414–419
Fuleihan GEH, Chen CJ, Rivkees SA, Marynick SP, Stock J, Pallotta JA, Brown EM (1989) Calcium-dependent release of N-terminal fragments and intact immunoreactive parathyroid hormone by human pathological parathyroid tissue in vitro. J Clin Endocrinol Metab 69:860–867
Gallacher SJ, Fraser WD, Logue FC, Dryburgh FJ, Cowan RA, Boyle IT, Ralston SH (1992) Factors predicting the acute effect of pamidronate on serum calcium in hypercalcemia of malignancy. Calcif Tissue Int 51:419–423
Gallacher SJ, Fraser WD, Farquharson MA, Logue FC, McArdle C, Boyle IT, Nairn ER, McNicol AM (1993) Coincidental occurrence of primary hyperparathyroidism and cancer associated hypercalcemia in a middle-aged man. Clin Endocrinol 38:433–437
Harms HM, Kaptaina U, Kuelpmann WR, Brabant G, Hesch RD (1989) Pulse amplitude and frequency modulation of parathyroid hormone in plasma. J Clin Endocrinol Metab 69:843–851
Herfarth K, Schmidt-Gayk H, Graf S, Maier A (1992) Circadian rhythm and pulsatility of parathyroid hormone secretion in man. Clin Endocrinol 37:511–519
Hollenberg AN, Arnold A (1991) Hypercalcemia with low-normal serum intact PTH: a novel presentation of primary hyperparathyroidism. Am J Med 91: 547–548
Husdan H, Rapoport A, Locke S (1973) Influence of posture on the serum concentration of calcium. Metabolism 22:787–797
Jacobus CH, Holick MF, Shao Q, Chen TC, Holm IA, Kolodny JM, Fuleihan GEH, Seely EW (1992) Hypervitaminosis D associated with drinking milk. N Engl J Med 326:1173–1177
Klee GG, Preissner CM, Schryver PG, Taylor RL, Kao PC (1992) Multisite immunochemiluminometric assay for simultaneously measuring whole-molecule and amino-terminal fragments of human parathyrin. Clin Chem 38:628–635
Krause U, Zielke A, Schmidt-Gayk H, Ehrenthal W, Beyer J (1989) Direct tubular effect on calcium retention by hydrochlorothiazide. J Endocrinol Invest 12: 531–535
LoCascio V, Adami S, Galvanini G, Ferrari M, Cominacini L, Tartarotti D (1985) Substrate-product relation of 1-hydroxylase activity in primary hyperparathyroidism. N Engl J Med 313:1123–1125
Ljunghall S, Joborn H, Roxin LE, Skarfors ET, Wide LE, Lithell HO (1988) Increase in serum parathyroid hormone after prolonged exercise. Med Sci Sports Exerc 20:122–125
Mallette LE, Khouri K, Zengotita H, Hollis BW, Malini S (1989) Lithium treatment increases intact and midregion parathyroid hormone and parathyroid volume. J Clin Endocrinol Metab 68:654–660
Marx SJ, Stock JL, Attie MF, Downs RW, Gardner DG, Brown EM, Spiegel AM, Doppman JL, Brennan MF (1980) Familial hypocalciuric hypercalcemia: recognition among patients referred after unsuccessful parathyroid exploration. Ann Intern Med 92:351–356
Marx SJ, Spiegel AM, Levine MA, Rizzoli RE, Lasker RD, Santora AC, Downs RW, Aurvach GD (1982) Familial hypocalciuric hypercalcemia, the relation to primary parathyroid hyperplasia. N Engl J Med 307:416–426

Marx SJ, Menczel J, Campbell G, Aurbach GD, Spiegel AM, Norton JA (1991) Heterogeneous size of the parathyroid glands in familial multiple endocrine neoplasia type 1. Clin Endocrinol 35:521–526

McElduff A, Lackmann M, Wilkinson M (1992) Antiidiotypic PTH antibodies as a cause of elevated immunoreactive parathyroid hormone in idiopathic hypoparathy roidism, a second case: another manifestation of autoimmune endocrine disease? Calcif Tissue Int 51:121–126

Meneghini LF, Oster JR, Camacho JR, Gkonos PJ, Roos BA (1993) Hypercalcemia in association with acute renal failure and rhabdomyolysis. Miner Electrolyte Metab 19:1–16

Nussbaum SR, Zahradnik RJ, Lavigne JR, Brennan GL, Nozawa-Ung K, Kim LY, Keutmann HT, Wang CA, Potts JTjr, Segre GV (1987) Highly sensitive two-site immunoradiometric assay of parathyrin, and its clinical utility in evaluating patients with hypercalcemia. Clin Chem 33:1364–1367

Palmer FJ, Nelson JC, Bacchus H (1974) The chloride-phosphate ratio in hypercalcemia. Ann Intern Med 80:200–204

Pandian MR, Morgan CH, Carlton E, Segre GV (1992) Modified immunoradiometric assay of parathyroid hormone-related protein: clinical application in the differential diagnosis of hypercalcemia. Clin Chem 38:282–288

Parfitt AM (1969) Chlorothiazide-induced hypercalcemia in juvenile osteoporosis and hyperparathyroidism. N Engl J Med 281:55–59

Paterson CR (1980) Vitamin-D poisoning: survey of causes in 21 patients with hypercalcemia. Lancet I:1164–1165

Payne RB, Carver ME, Morgan DB (1979) Interpretation of serum total calcium: effects of adjustment for albumin concentration on frequency of abnormal values and on detection of change in the individual. J Clin Pathol 32:56–60

Reeves CD, Palmer F, Bacchus H, Longerbeam JK (1975) Differential diagnosis of hypercalcemia by the chloride/phosphate ratio. Am J Surg 130:166–171

Rosenthal N, Insogna KL, Godsall JW, Smaldone L, Waldron JA, Stewart AF (1985) Elevations in circulating 1,25-dihydroxyvitamin D in three patients with lymphoma-associated hypercalcemia. J Clin Endocrinol Metab 60:29–33

Schilling T, Pecherstorfer M, Blind E, Leidig G, Ziegler R, Raue F (1993) Parathyroid hormone-related protein (PTHrP) does not regulate 1,25-dihydroxyvitamin D serum levels in hypercalcemia of malignancy. J Clin Endocrinol Metab 76: 801–803

Schmidt-Gayk H, Stengel R, Haueisen H, Huefner M, Ritz E, Jakobs KH (1977) Hyperparathyroidism: influence of glomerular filtration rate on urinary excretion of cyclic AMP. Klin Wschr 55:275–281

Schmidt-Gayk H, Radeck H, Haerdt H (1991) Erfassung von Stoerungen des Calcium- und Phosphatstoffwechsels, der Nierenfunktion und der Ernaehrung: Programm für IBM-kompatible Personal-Computer. Nieren Hochdruckkrankht 20:678–684

Segre V (1990) Advances in techniques for measurement of parathyroid hormone, current applications in clinical medicine and directions for future research. Trends Endocrinol Metab (TEM) 243–247

Seelig MS (1970) Hyperreactivity to vitamin D. Med Counterpoint 2:28–44

Shane E (1993) Hypercalcemia: pathogenesis, clinical manifestations, and differential diagnosis. In: Favus MJ (ed) Primer on the metabolic bone diseases and disorders of mineral metabolism, 2nd edn. Raven, New York, pp 153–155

Shaw NJ, Wheeldon J, Brocklebank JT (1992) The tubular maximum for calcium reabsorption: a normal range in children. Clin Endocrinol 36:193–195

Solal MEC, Sebert JL, Boudailliez B, Marie A, Moriniere P, Gueris J, Bouillon R, Fournier A (1991) Comparison of intact, midregion, and carboxy terminal assays of parathyroid hormone for the diagnosis of bone disease in hemodialyzed patients. J Clin Endocrinol Metab 73:516–524

Streeten EA, Weinstein LS, Norton JA, Mulvihill JJ, White BJ, Friedman E, Jaffe G, Brandi ML, Stewart K, Zimering MB, Spiegel AM, Aurbach GD, Marx SJ (1992) Studies in a kindred with parathyroid carcinoma. J Clin Endocrinol Metab 75:362–366

Szabo J, Khosla S, Heath HIII (1993) Familial hyperparathyroid syndromes. In: Favus MJ (ed) Primer on the metabolic bone diseases and disorders of mineral metabolism, 2nd edn. Raven, New York, pp 164–166

Thome JF, Bilezikian JP, Clemens TL, Silverberg SJ, Shane E, Lindsay R (1990) Suppression of parathyroid hormone secretion with oral calcium in normal subjects and patients with primary hyperparathyroidism. J Clin Endocrinol Metab 70: 951–956

Vieth R (1990) The mechanisms of vitamin D toxicity. Bone Miner 11:267–272

Vosik WM, Anderson CF, Steffee WP, Johnson WJ, Arnaud CD, Goldsmith RS (1972) Successful medical management of osteitis fibrosa due to "tertiary" hyperparathyroidism. Mayo Clin Proc 47:110–113

Wilkinson M, McElduff A, Wilson J, Haber P, Freeman A, Robertson M, Mathews P (1990) Spontaneously occurring antibodies to parathyroid hormone. J Clin Endocrinol Metab 70:1744–1749

Yoshimoto K, Yamasaki R, Sakai H, Tezuka U, Takahashi M, Iizuka M, Sekiya T, Saito S (1989) Ectopic production of parathyroid hormone by small cell lung cancer in a patient with hypercalcemia. J Clin Endocrinol Metab 68:976–981

Drug Therapy of Hypercalcemia Due to Malignancy

F. Raue[1] and M. Pecherstorfer[2]

[1] Department of Internal Medicine I – Endocrinology and Metabolism, University of Heidelberg, Bergheimerstraße 58, 69115 Heidelberg, Germany
[2] Department of Internal Medicine I – Oncology, Wilhelminen Hospital, Montleartstraße 37, 1171 Vienna, Austria

Introduction

Hypercalcemia is a serious complication of a number of malignant and benign disorders. The two most common causes of severe hypercalcemia are cancer and primary hyperparathyroidism. The differential diagnosis between cancer-related hypercalcemia and primary hyperparathyroidism is made by measuring intact parathyroid hormone (PTH). While most patients with primary hyperparathyroidism have elevated levels of intact PTH in their serum, in virtually all patients with hypercalcemia of malignancy the levels are suppressed (Blind et al. 1990; Nussbaum et al. 1987). Hypercalcemia in patients with cancer is usually due to secretion of parathyroid hormone-related protein (PTHrP) by the tumor. Assays for PTHrP are now available, and hypercalcemia of malignancy can be confirmed by an elevated level of serum PTHrP in the majority of patients (Blind et al. 1992). Other and rare causes of hypercalcemia of malignancy are the secretion of other bone-resorbing substances by the tumor, such as 1,25-dihydroxyvitamin D, or local effects of osteolytic bone metastases (Rosol and Capen 1992; Martin and Grill 1992). The clinical features of hypercalcemia can range from asymptomatic to severe intractable nausea and vomiting, dehydration, coma, and death. In general, the severity of the signs and symptoms is proportional to the degree of hypercalcemia and is also influenced by the degree of dehydration (Bajorunas 1990).

The ideal treatment for patients with cancer-related hypercalcemia is tumor ablation whether by surgery, radiation, or chemotherapy directed against the underlying malignancy (Bilezikian 1992). For the vast majority of patients, however, this is unrealistic, since most have advanced disease and have failed to respond to primary cytotoxic therapy. Therefore, symptomatic medical management of hypercalcemia is recommended: correction of dehydration, enhancement of renal excretion of calcium, inhibition of accelerated bone resorption, and inhibition of absorption of calcium from the gut (Table 1) (Bilezikian 1992; Moskilde et al. 1991; Ritch 1990). The

Table 1. Management of hypercalcemia of malignancy

Therapy of primary disease
Tumor ablation (surgical, radiation, cytotoxic)
Restoration of extracellular fluid volume (rehydration)
Saline infusion
Enhancement of urinary calcium excretion
Saline infusion plus furosemide
Inhibition of bone resorption
Bisphosphonates (clodronate, pamidronate)
Calcitonin
Glucocorticoids
Plicamycin (mithramycin)
Gallium nitrate
Prostaglandin synthetase inhibitors
WR-2721
Reduction of intestinal calcium absorption
Low calcium diet
Glucocorticoids
Others
Dialysis
Mobilization

choice of therapy depends on the presence of hypercalcemic symptoms and the levels of serum calcium. Patients with mild hypercalcemia who are asymptomatic (serum calcium level usually less than 3.0 mmol/l) can be treated with the nonurgent form of therapy. Severe hypercalcemia (serum calcium more than 3.5 mmol/l) requires immediate and effective therapy, since it can be self-perpetuating and is potentially fatal. In patients with malignancy, hypercalcemia is usually a manifestation of advanced disease which is likely to be fatal in the near future. Indeed, no controlled trial has demonstrated a survival advantage for any hypercalcemia-directed therapy (Ralston et al. 1990). In many of these patients judgement is made to forego life-sustaining treatment. Sometimes the better part of valor is not to treat the hypercalcemia at all. In such patients, hypercalcemia can provide sedation and analgesia which can decrease and abbreviate suffering (Attie 1989).

Pathophysiological Considerations

The principal source of excess extracellular calcium in hypercalcemia of malignancy is enhanced bone resorption. Three types of hypercalcemia have been described: (1) humoral hypercalcemia of malignancy, defined as hypercalcemia occurring without evidence of bone metastases and mediated by humoral factors; (2) hypercalcemia apparently due to direct osteolysis by bone metastases; and (3) hypercalcemia of hematological tumors, which is mediated by different humoral factors (Mundy and Martin 1992). The distinctions between the three types are becoming less and less clear, since recent studies have established the essential role of PTHrP in all three types of hypercalcemia of malignancy.

Despite the homology between PTH and PTHrP, different effects on bone, intestine and kidney have been observed. In bone a negative balance due to increased bone resorption and profound depression of bone formation develops in most patients with humoral hypercalcemia of malignancy. In contrast to patients with hyperparathyroidism the number of osteoclasts is not increased. This could also be confirmed by measuring the level of bone GLA protein (osteocalcin), a biochemical marker of osteoblasts. Osteocalcin was generally elevated in hyperparathyroid patients but not in patients with hypercalcemia of malignancy (Delmas et al. 1986). Bone formation thus appears to be reduced in patients with hypercalcemia of malignancy by "uncoupling" of osteoclastic and osteoblastic activities.

Intestinal calcium absorption is generally suppressed in patients with hypercalcemia of malignancy, as 1,25-dihydroxyvitamin D levels are generally low (Stewart et al. 1980). In primary hyperparathyroidism the production of 1,25-dihydroxyvitamin D is most often increased (Mosekilde et al. 1989), while in patients with hypercalcemia of malignancy PTHrP levels are increased and 1,25-dihydroxyvitamin D levels are usually suppressed (Schilling et al. 1993; Stewart et al. 1980). In some patients with malignant lymphomas, hypercalcemia is due to the production of 1,25-dihydroxyvitamin D (Breslau et al. 1984). Here, the increased circulating levels of 1,25-dihydroxyvitamin D cause hypercalcemia by both enhanced intestinal calcium absorption and bone resorption.

The role of the kidney in hypercalcemia of malignancy is complex. Although there is an increase in tubular resorption of calcium, resulting from the specific renal effect of PTHrP, there is, nonetheless, a decrease in the glomerular filtration rate, resulting from the contracted circulating volume. PTHrP, autonomously secreted by many tumors, enhances renal tubular calcium reabsorption similar to PTH in primary hyperparathyroidism. The ability of the kidney to excrete the increased filtered load of calcium is impaired in patients with hypercalcemia of malignancy (Bonjour et al. 1988; Percival et al. 1985; Ralston et al. 1984). Hypercalcemia and hypercalciuria impair renal sodium and water reabsorption, which causes polyuria and dehydration. Associated nausea and vomiting further exacerbate volume contraction. Volume contraction of the extracellular fluid reduces the glomerular filtration rate and thereby renal excretion of calcium. This, in turn, leads to a further rise in the level of serum calcium (Fig. 1). The development of nephrocalcinosis and reduced blood flow further perpetuate this vicious cycle.

In general, hypercalcemia develops when the entry of calcium from bone into the extracellular fluid overwhelms the renal mechanisms that normally maintain serum calcium within a narrow range. To be maximally effective, therapy for hypercalcemia must be based on the pathogenetic mechanism

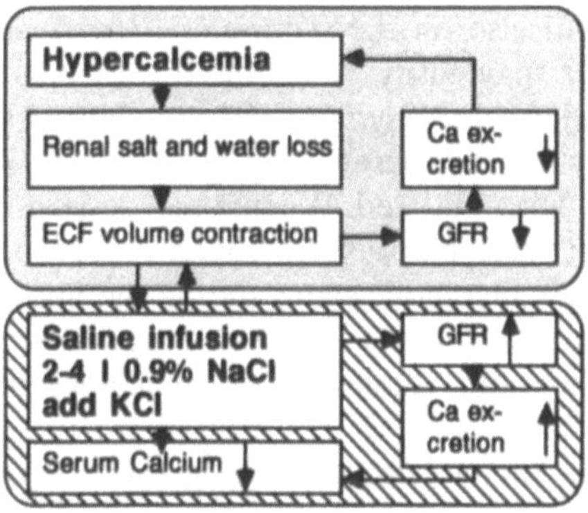

Fig. 1. Role of the kidney in the development of hypercalcemia and the therapeutic approach to stop the vicious circle. *ECF*, extracellular fluid; *GFR*, glomerular filtration rate

involved, including correction of dehydration, enhancement of renal excretion of calcium, inhibition of accelerated bone resorption and treatment of the underlying disorder.

Treatment of Hypercalcemia

Therapeutic Options

In cancer-related hypercalcemia the best treatment is clearly that which inhibits or ablates the underlying malignancy. Unfortunately, this is often not possible, as only a minority of patients have a tumor that is curable by primary resection, and frequently hypercalcemia occurs in the presence of recurrent and progressive disseminated disease that has become refractory to standard antineoplastic therapy. There is no widespread agreement on the indication for medical management of hypercalcemia of malignancy. When the patient has an incurable, widely disseminated cancer for which no specific therapy is contemplated, less aggressive or even on specific antihypercalcemic treatment may be appropriate. The decision will depend on the severity of the hypercalcemia and the previous, current, and expected quality of life of the patient, which itself will depend on whether any further effective treatment of the malignancy is thought possible. The decision to treat with specific measures must be given careful consideration in each case.

Some authors believe that all patients with hypercalcemia should be treated, because serum calcium levels tend to rise in a steadily progressive manner (Mundy 1990b). Others have claimed that a therapeutic decision, especially in patients with moderate hypercalcemia, should be based not only on the serum calcium concentration but also on the symptoms (Bilezikian 1992). The symptoms of hypercalcemia may easily be confused with those occurring late in the course of advanced cancer. Asymptomatic patients with mild hypercalcemia may require only careful observation, particularly if cytotoxic therapy for the malignancy is being initiated. When tumor response is expected to occur slowly, specific antihypercalcemic therapy may be initially required to stabilize the patient's metabolic status during the initial staging evaluation and start of treatment (Ritch 1990). This includes adequate fluid and salt intake, control of nausea and vomiting, and avoidance of immobilization.

Severe symptomatic hypercalcemia or serum calcium greater than 3.5 mmol/l is a metabolic emergency requiring immediate intervention, independent of the cause of the hypercalcemia, to improve the condition of the patient and to provide time for further evaluation. This calcium value is based on the assumption that the serum albumin concentration is normal, but in patients with severe hypercalcemia the serum calcium concentration may be elevated because of dehydration or reduced albumin levels due to chronic illness. A well-accepted correction factor is to add to the measured total serum calcium 0.02 mmol/l per gram albumin lower than 40 g/l (Shane 1990). Restoration of extracellular fluid volume by saline hydration, induction of calciuria, and inhibition of bone resorption by antihypercalcemic agents are the necessary measures for immediate therapy of hypercalcemia. Lowering the serum calcium is sometimes of significant palliative value, especially since it ameliorates gastrointestinal and neurologic symptoms.

General Management

Hydration

Extracellular volume expansion is an essential component of any therapeutic program to restore adequate hydration and increase renal calcium output (Fig. 1). The continuous intravenous administration of isotonic saline is the first step in managing severe hypercalcemia. Administration of 2–4 l of 0.9% sodium chloride solution over the first 24–48 h will restore intravascular volume, thereby correcting the hemoconcentration, and will increase renal calcium clearance. The increase in glomerular filtration rate leads to an increase in filtration of calcium such that proximal sodium and calcium reabsorption are decreased. The increase in sodium and water excretion increases the calciuresis. The rate of administration of saline should be based on the severity of hypercalcemia, the extent of dehydration, and the ability of the patient's cardiovascular system to tolerate volume expansion. In the past, very large volumes of fluids were infused, often combined with large quantities of furosemide. The patients required intensive monitoring to avoid fluid overload, but complete correction of hypercalcemia was rarely observed (Hosking et al. 1981). For this reason, and because of the advent of effective hypocalcemic drugs, much lower volumes are now infused.

Frequent measurements of plasma electrolytes are made, initially twice daily, as hypokalemia is frequently present prior to treatment or develops during treatment. This is of special importance in patients taking digitalis preparations, since the combined effect of digitalis, hypercalcemia, hypokalemia, and hypomagnesemia on the myocardium is synergistic and may lead to fatal arrhythmias. An appropriate intravenous potassium supplement should be given. Urine output must be maintained to avoid possible fluid overload. Oral intake of fluids should be encouraged if the patient is not nauseous or vomiting. In general, there is a modest decrease in the concentration of serum calcium as a result of dilutional effects and enhanced urinary calcium excretion; since hypercalcemia is, in most cases, associated with increased bone resorption, serum calcium will again begin to rise; however, the serum calcium level seldom normalizes except in those patients with only mild hypercalcemia (Hosking et al. 1981; Singer 1991).

Diuretics

Loop diuretics such as furosemide or ethacrynic acid have been shown to induce calciuresis by inhibiting calcium and sodium reabsorption in the ascending limb of the loop of Henle (Suki et al. 1970). Routine use of loop diuretics may be harmful, unless their administration is delayed until volume expansion is achieved. In volume-contracted patients these potent diuretics can enhance fluid loss, potentially reduce calcium clearance, and raise the level of serum calcium. Thiazide diuretics are not indicated in the situation of volume deficit since they enhance tubular reabsorption of calcium and thus may actually exacerbate hypercalcemia.

Intensive administration of furosemide (80–100 mg every 2–4 h with large amounts of fluid) is a problematic but effective regimen for severe hypercalcemia (Suki et al. 1970). All patients treated in this manner should be in an intensive care unit with a central venous line placed to avoid volume overload or depletion. This approach may be particularly dangerous for patients with impaired myocardial function. It should be noted that the increasing availability of potent antiresorptive agents makes this heroic form of therapy unnecessary in most patients. Instead, more moderate doses (20–40 mg every 12 h) of furosemide are given to prevent fluid overload. This precaution is particularly important in older patients whose cardiovascular status may be marginal.

Clinical improvement usually occurs after rehydration over 24–48 h. However, normalization of serum calcium seldom occurs, except in very mild hypercalcemia. Other therapy is usually required, especially inhibition of excessive mobilization of calcium from bone.

Bisphosphonates

Chemistry and Action

Although Eilon and Mundy (1978) demonstrated that tumor cells have the capacity to resorb bone directly, the osteoclasts are usually the mediators of neoplastic bone destruction. They are stimulated by tumor cell derived cytokines and prostaglandins in a paracrine or endocrine way (Garrett et al. 1987b; Greaves et al. 1980; Ibbotson et al. 1985; Powell et al. 1991; Shirakawa et al. 1988). Bisphosphonates strongly inhibit osteoclast-mediated bone resorption. Thus, they have been used in the treatment of benign and malignant bone diseases since the early 1970s (Douglas et al. 1983; Elomaa et al. 1983; Jacobs et al. 1981; Russell et al. 1974). Bisphosphonates are also important as bone avid carrier for Tc-99m in radiopharmaceutical bone imaging, where an increased uptake of the radiolabeled bisphosphonate is found in areas of active bone formation (Fogelman and McKillop 1991; Pecherstorfer et al. 1993a). The theoretical background of bisphosphonates has been reviewed in an issue of *Recent Results in Cancer Research* (Fleisch 1989). Therefore, we want to confine our remarks to the clinical use of bisphosphonates in the treatment of hypercalcemia of malignancy, following a short presentation of different bisphosphonates, of their specific characteristics and of their mechanism of action.

Bisphosphonates are derivatives of the physiologically occurring pyrophosphoric acid. They are characterized by a central phosphorus-carbon-phosphorus structure, which, in contrast to the phosphorus-oxygen-phosphorus structure of pyrophosphoric acid, cannot be degraded by the serum phosphates (Fleisch 1989). At present, three generations of bisphosphonates can be differentiated, mainly by their activity in inhibiting bone resorption and their effects on the calcification of normal bone. Etidronate (1-hydroxyethylene-1,1-bisphosphonic acid) was the first bisphosphonate examined in clinical trials and the substance most extensively used. The long-term oral administration of etidronate has been associated with demineralization of normal bone (Guncaga et al. 1974) and with spontaneous fractures (Reiner et al. 1980). Bisphosphonates of the second and third generation lack the demineralizing effect on normal bone. Second-generation bisphosphonates are clodronate (dichloromethylene-bisphosphonic acid), tiludronate (chloro-4-phentylthiomethylidene-bisphosphonic acid), and pamidronate (3-amino-1-hydroxypropylidene-1,1-bisphosphonic acid), the first aminobisphosphonate. In a rat model, clodronate and tiludronate display an antiresorbing potency 10 times higher than etidronate, whereas pamidronate is about 100 times more effective. A third generation of bisphosphonates is represented by the aminoderivatives alendronate (4-amino-1-hydroxybutilidene bisphosphonic acid) and BM 21.0955 [1-hydroxy-3 (methylpenthylamino)-propylidene-bisphosphonic acid], which are about 1000 and 10000 times more effective than etidronate in inhibiting bone resorption. The relative activities of the different bisphosphonates demonstrated in the rat appear to be also repesentative for their bone-protecting potencies in humans (Fleisch 1991; Mühlbauer et al. 1991).

The exact mechanism of the action of bisphosphonates is still unknown. However, it is clear that the first step in influencing the osteoclast activity is the rapid chemisorption of bisphosphonates to the osseous surface. Various effects have been described following the ingestion of bisphosphonate-impregnated bone by osteoclasts: a decrease in the total number of osteoclasts (Evans et al. 1982; Flanagan and Chambers 1989; Frijlink et al. 1979), an increase of partially irregular shaped cells (De Vernejoul et al. 1987; Marie et al. 1985; Miller et al. 1977), an increase or a decrease in dependency of the administered dose (Mühlbauer et al. 1991) or an early increase followed by the reduction of the osteoclasts (Marshall et al. 1990). Besides the direct toxic effect on mature osteoclasts, Boonekamp et al. (1988) also described an impairment of the recruitment of osteoclast-precursor cells by the bisphosphonate therapy.

Clinical Use

Bisphosphonates have been used in a great variety of schedules and dosages in the treatment of hypercalcemia of malignancy (Table 2). In clinical trials pamidronate appeared to be more effective than etidronate in restoring normocalcemia (Gucalp et al. 1992). In a randomized study, Ralston et al. (1989) compared etidronate, clodronate and pamidronate. They observed normalization of serum calcium in 14 of 16 patients treated with pamidronate compared to 6 of 16 patients in the clodronate group and 5 of 16 patients in the etidronate group. These results have given cause for discussion since the dose of clodronate administered (600 mg i.v. on day 0) was relatively low (Kanis et al. 1990).

When the intravenous route was chosen, usually more than 70% of the patients treated with clodronate or pamidronate showed a transient normalization of the serum calcium levels. Since bisphosphonates lower serum calcium by affecting the osteoclast activity and do not influence renal calcium handling, hypercalcemic patients with raised circulating parathyroid hormone-related protein (PTHrP) display a reduced response rate when compared to cases with low or undetectable PTHrP (Blind et al. 1992; Body et al. 1993; Dodwell et al. 1991; Gurney et al. 1993). Thiébaud et al. (1988) demonstrated that an increase in the dose of the bisphosphonates leads to a higher response rate and to a longer duration of the response. If the hypercalcemia relapses, bisphosphonates are effective again in decreasing serum calcium. However, a smaller proportion of the patients become normocalcemic if the bisphosphonate treatment is repeated in the original dosage (Thiébaud et al. 1990). Escalating the dose of the bisphosphonate (e.g., up to 180 mg pamidronate as a single day infusion) can restore

Table 2. Schedules, dosages and responses of bisphosphonates in the treatment of tumor-associated hypercalcemia

Authors	Year	Bisphosphonates	Number of patients	Dosage and schedule	Normal calcium[a]
Jacobs et al.	1981	Clodronate	12	2.5–5.0 mg/kg body wt. i.v.[b]	91%
Paterson	1983	Clodronate	19	800–3200 mg p.o.	78%
Harinck	1987	Pamidronate	132	15 mg i.v.[b]	90%
Thiébaud et al.	1988	Pamidronate	52	30–90 mg i.v., day 0	82%
Gurney	1989	Pamidronate	15	30–90 mg i.v., day 0[c]	46%
Ziegler	1989	Clodronate	34	300 mg i.v.[b]	82%
Dumon	1991	Tiludronate	19	3.0–6.0 mg/kg body wt. i.v.; day 0–day 2	72%
Pecherstorfer	1991	Pamidronate	28	30–60 mg i.v.; day 0[c,d]	100%
Blind et al.	1992	BM-210955	10	0.2–1.6 mg i.v.; day 0	40%
Gucalp et al.	1992	Etidronate	34	7.5 mg/kg body wt. i.v.; day 0–day 2	41%
		Pamidronate	30	60 mg i.v.; day 0	70%
Zysset	1992	Alendronate	10	10 mg i.v.–2 h[e]	70%
			10	10 mg i.v.–24 h[e]	90%
O'Rourke	1993	Clodronate	30	1500 mg i.v.; day 0	80%

[a] Proportion of patients with at least transient normalization of serum calcium.
[b] Daily administration until normalization of serum calcium.
[c] Adapted to the serum calcium level.
[d] Treatment was repeated if the serum calcium level was $\geqslant$2.8 mmol/l on day 3.
[e] Duration of infusion.

normocalcemia in patients with a second or third relapse of hypercalcemia and previous resistance to bisphosphonate treatment (Pecherstorfer and Thièbaud 1992).

The most important adverse effect of bisphosphonate treatment is the potential nephrotoxicity, which appears to be caused by the formation and dropout of bisphosphonate-calcium complexes (Bounameaux et al. 1983). This problem usually does not arise when the drug is not injected but infuses over a period of one to several hours dependent on the dose administered. In a proportion of the patients treated with pamidronate, a transient increase in the body temperature can be demonstrated, which usually does not exceed 1°C and subsides within 24 h. However, some patients experience fever up to 40°C. This acute phase reaction appears to be mediated by the release of tumor necrosis factor alpha and is associated with the expression of CD 69, an early activation marker on T lymphocytes (Pecherstorfer et al. 1993c).

Changes in Laboratory Parameters

Raised serum calcium levels suppress the secretion of PTH (Conlin et al. 1989). Decreasing serum calcium induces an elevation of the serum concentrations of PTH, which can exceed the upper limit of normal range (Body et al. 1992; Grill et al. 1992; Papapoulos et al. 1986; Pecherstorfer et al. 1993a). This secondary hyperparathyroidism is associated with an increase in the initially suppressed levels of 1,25-dihydroxyvitamin D (Papapoulos et al. 1986; Schilling et al. 1993). Moreover, due to its phosphaturic effect it might be the cause of the transient fall in serum phosphate (Papapoulos et al. 1986; Thiébaud et al. 1988).

Usually, a significant decrease in serum creatinine can also be observed reflecting the improved rehydration after the restoration of normocalcemia. The serum concentrations of PTHrP are obviously not influenced by the course of serum calcium (Blind et al. 1992; Body et al. 1993; Grill et al. 1992; Pecherstorfer et al. 1992; Schilling et al. 1993).

Treatment of tumor-induced hypercalcemia with bisphosphonates leads to an impressive reduction in the urinary excretion of calcium, of hydroxyproline and of the pyridinium crosslinks pyridinoline and deoxypyridinoline, reflecting the inhibition of bone resorption (Fig. 2) (Body and Delmas 1992; Pecherstorfer et al. 1993b; Ralston et al. 1989; Thiébaud et al. 1988).

Calcitonin

Calcitonin, a peptide derived from the C cells of the thyroid, acts on bone to inhibit osteoclastic resorption and on the kidney to promote urinary calcium excretion. In theory, this hormone should be an ideal agent in the control

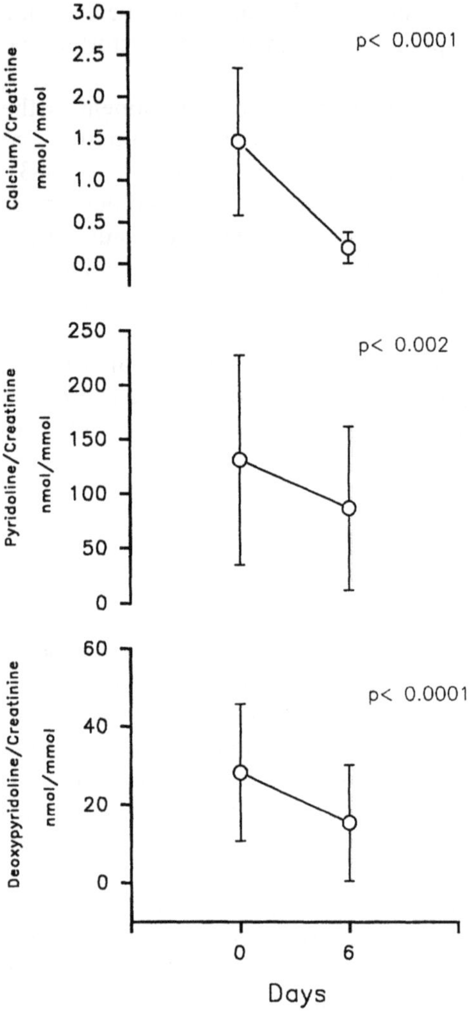

Fig. 2. Changes in the urinary excretion of calcium and of the pyridinium crosslinks pyridinoline and deoxypyridinoline (mean ± SD) following treatment of malignancy-associated hypercalcemia with bisphosphonates. Thirty-nine patients with tumor-associated hypercalcemia (mean serum calcium on day 0: 3.08 ± 0.31 mmol/l) were treated with pamidronate (30–60 mg) or BM 21.0955 (0.6–2.0 mg) on day 0. On day 6, the mean serum calcium concentration was 2.39 ± 0.35 mmol/l. The fall in serum calcium level was paralleled by a dectease in the calcium/creatinine ratio (day 0: 1.46 ± 0.87 mmol/mmol vs. day 6: 0.20 ± 0.18 mmol/mmol), of the pyridinoline/creatinine ratio (day 0: 129.04 ± 82.63 nmol/mmol vs. day 6: 93.41 ± 62.48 nmlo/mmol) and of the deoxypyridinoline/creatinine ratio (day 0: 27.0 ± 15.9 nmol/mmol vs. day 6: 15.61 ± 11.78 nmol/mmol). In our laboratory the upper limit of the normal range for the calcium/creatinine ratio is 0.25 mmol/mmol, for the pyridinoline/creatinine ratio 54 nmol/mmol and for the deoxypyridinoline/creatinine ratio 12.5 nmol/mmol

of excessive bone resorption (Hosking and Gilson 1984). The major advantages are its rapid onset of action and its safe use in patients with dehydration and renal insufficiency. Side effects are generally mild and may include nausea, abdominal cramps, vomiting and flushing. Reduction of serum calcium can be observed within a few hours after calcitonin administration (Silva and Becker 1973; Wisneski 1990), but the effect appears to be of brief duration, as serum calcium increases, despite continued calcitonin administration, within 48 h (Binstock and Mundy 1980; Warrell et al. 1988). Most patients treated with calcitonin alone show only a transient response, a phenomenon that also has been observed in vitro and has been referred to as the "escape phenomenon."

Calcitonin is usually administered subcutaneously or intramuscularly in a dose of 4–8 U/kg body wt. every 6–12 h. Nasal and rectal administration of calcitonin has also been reported (Dumon et al. 1992; Thiébaud et al. 1990). In 21 patients treated with calcitonin, the mean serum calcium fell from 3.45 to 3.16 mmol/l within 48 h. Ten of the patients, however, showed little or no response (Hosking and Gilson 1984).

Glucocorticoids have been shown to prevent the escape from calcitonin's inhibition of bone resorption in vitro (Raisz et al. 1972). Administration of glucocorticoids in combination with calcitonin has been explored in hypercalcemic cancer patients in three studies (Binstock and Mundy 1980; Hosking et al. 1990; Ralston et al. 1985) and was shown to be more effective than either agent alone. However, in both series only 4 of 24 patients had a serum calcium level in the normal range during treatment. Also, periodic withdrawal of calcitonin has been recommended to permit prolonged maintenance therapy with the combination (Hosking et al. 1981). However, this approach has not been widely accepted. Furthermore, prolonged steroid use may be associated with undesirable adverse effects. This combination was not more effective than pamidronate or plicamycin in one study (Ralston et al. 1985). Combined bisphosphonate and calcitonin therapy has been reported to be more efficacious (Ralston et al. 1985) than bisphosphonate therapy alone (Fatemi et al. 1992; Thiébaud et al. 1990).

Despite the fact that calcitonin is relatively short-acting and an only moderately effective agent, it has a role in the treatment of hypercalcemia as an adjunctive drug. In patients with severe hypercalcemia and renal insufficiency, in whom immediate therapy is necessary, calcitonin will induce the most rapid (but moderate) decrease in serum calcium levels. This is acceptable while waiting for the therapeutic effect of slower-acting but more potent agents such as bisphosphonates.

Plicamycin (Mithramycin)

Mithramycin was isolated from *Streptomyces plicatus* (plicamycin) and belongs to the group of antibiotics with cytostatic activity. Mithramycin is an inhibitor of DNA-directed RNA synthesis (Yabro et al. 1965). It is active against testicular cancer and exerts a hypocalcemic effect by irreversibly damaging the osteoclasts (Brown and Kennedy 1965). It has to be administered strictly intravenously. Besides acute nausea and vomiting its use is associated marked thrombocytopenia and with renal, hepatic and neurologic toxicity (Chabner 1993; Ralston et al. 1985; Thürlimann et al. 1992). Doses of 25 μg/kg body weight or a total dose of 1.5–2.0 mg given as an infusion over 4 h are recommended (Mundy 1990b; Warrell 1993). Twenty-four to 48 h after the administration of the drug, a rapid decrease in serum calcium can be observed. In the literature, the number of hypercalcemic patients responding to mithramycin treatment with a normalization of serum calcium varies between 45% and 80% (Mundy et al. 1983; Thürlimann et al. 1992). Occasionally, a rapid increase in serum calcium to hypercalcemic levels can be observed in initially responding patients (Mundy et al. 1983). If hypercalcemia relapses, mithramycin therapy can be successfully repeated but close monitoring of platelet count and kidney and liver function is essential. Due to its side effects treatment of tumor-associated hypercalcemia with mithramycin should only be considered after therapy with maximally tolerated doses of bisphosphonates has failed to normalize serum calcium (Bonjour and Rizzoli 1992).

Gallium Nitrate

Gallium nitrate is a new antineoplastic compound that inhibits bone resorption and causes hypocalcemia as an adverse effect (Todd and Fitton 1991). Gallium nitrate acts directly on bone, both inhibiting bone resorption by reducing the solubility of bone crystals (Bockman 1991) and affecting osteoclast and osteoblast activity (Guidon et al. 1993). In clinical studies performed in patients with hypercalcemia of malignancy, gallium nitrate has had significant effects (Warrell et al. 1986, 1987, 1988). Normalization of serum calcium is accompanied by a reduction in the urinary excretion of hydroxyproline, confirming its action as an inhibitor of bone resorption (Warrell et al. 1987). The drug is approved to be given as a continuous intravenous infusion for 5 days at a dose of 200 mg/m^2 per day. Normocalcemia was found in more than 75% of patients treated with 5-day gallium nitrate infusions compared to 27% of patients treated with calcitonin (Warrell et al. 1988); the duration of response was also significantly longer with gallium (median 11 vs. 2 days). In another study comparing gallium nitrate and etidronate, normalization of serum calcium was achieved in 82% of patients receiving gallium and in 43% of those receiving etidronate (Warrell et al. 1991). Nephrotoxicity is a potential adverse effect of the drug. Although gallium nitrate is a promising therapeutic agent for treating hypercalcemia, clinical experience with it is still quite limited.

Glucocorticoids

Since the introduction of the bisphosphonates, the use of corticosteroids has been more and more restricted to the treatment of hypercalcemia in hematological neoplasms: hypercalcemia can be frequently demonstrated in multiple myeloma and adult T-cell lymphoma but it rarely occurs in Hodgkin's disease, B-cell lymphoma or acute leukemia (Bunn et al. 1983; Mundy 1990a). The most important pathophysiological mechanisms leading to hypercalcemia in these entities are the release of lymphotoxin (multiple myeloma) or parathyroid hormone-related protein (adult T-cell lymphoma) and the conversion of 25-hydroxyvitamin D to 1,25-dihydroxyvitamin D by the tumor cells (adult T-cell lymphomas and other lymphatic neoplasms) (Garrett et al. 1987; Motokura et al. 1989; Rosenthal et al. 1985). Glucocorticoids lower the serum calcium level by exerting cytotoxic effects on lymphatic cells (thus reducing the release of osteoclast-stimulating cytokines), by inhibiting the action of vitamin D and by reducing the gastrointestinal resorption of calcium (Attie 1989). A daily dose of 60–100 mg prednisone is recommended to control hypercalcemia (Warrell 1993). However, as far as we know, a prospective trial evaluating the hypocalcemic effect of glucocorticoid treatment (without chemotherapy) in a large number of patients with hematological neoplasms has never been performed. Thus, exact information concerning the response rate is not available.

Despite the finding that corticosteroids downregulate the expression of PTHrP by carcinoma cell lines in vitro (Ikeda et al. 1989; Kasono et al. 1991; Lu et al. 1989), they exert hardly any calcium-lowering effect in hypercalcemia associated with solid tumors. Percival et al. (1984) compared the course of serum calcium in 15 hypercalcemic patients with various carcinomas treated with fluid repletion and prednisolone (20–60 mg daily by mouth) to 13 patients who had only received rehydration therapy. He could not show any benefit of adding corticosteroids.

Miscellaneous Compounds

The radio- and chemoprotective compound WR-2721 suppresses PTH secretion, directly inhibits bone resorption, and interferes with renal tubular calcium reabsorption (Glover et al. 1983). Hypocalcemia was observed as an adverse effect during initial clinical studies; further studies demonstrated activity in treating hypercalcemia of malignancy, including that caused by parathyroid carcinoma (Glover et al. 1985). After an acute infusion there is only a moderate and brief reduction in serum calcium. There have been no clinical trials with this agent in hypercalcemic patients to assess its efficiency and safety during long-term administration.

The serum calcium concentration can be dramatically lowered by intravenous infusion of sodium phosphate by raising the calcium phosphate ion product above the solubility product, thus driving calcium into tissue. Potential organ damage from calcium phosphate precipitation in tissues such as lungs, heart, and kidney (where it can cause acute renal failure) severely limits the use of phosphate infusion in the treatment of hypercalcemia (Shackney and Hasson 1967; Vernava et al. 1987). It should therefore be restricted to patients with extreme life-threatening hypercalcemia in whom all other measures have failed. In patients with severe renal failure and hypercalcemia, dialysis with a low-calcium dialysate is very effective in lowering the serum calcium concentration (Cardella et al. 1979), but the effect is of short duration. In this situation volume expansion will be less effective in eliminating calcium, calcitonin can still be used, and bisphosphonates (reduced dose) are likely to be effective. Prostaglandins have been postulated to be mediators of bone resorption in malignancy-associated hypercalcemia. Initial reports suggested that prostaglandin synthetase inhibitors such as aspirin and indomethacin could correct hypercalcemia in patients with a variety of cancers (Seyberth et al. 1975). However, subsequent studies have shown that these drugs are rarely effective (Benner et al. 1982).

It may seem logical to reduce calcium intake. It is, however, difficult to recommend a diet with a low calcium content, which at the same time is palatable and sufficient in energy. Generally, absorption of calcium in the gut is reduced in patients with cancer and hypercalcemia due to regulatory mechanisms, nausea and vomiting (Coombs et al. 1976), and suppressed 1,25-dihydroxyvitamin D levels. Reduction of dietary calcium intake in patients with hypercalcemia of malignancy is therefore of little benefit. Only in patients with high levels of 1,25-dihydroxyvitamin D, for example, such as occurs in lymphoma, could reduction of calcium intake be beneficial.

As hypercalcemia and hypercalciuria are complications in immobilized patients with enhanced bone turnover, immobilization may contribute to the hypercalcemia observed in patients with malignant disease. The best way to treat these patients is to let them return to the weight-bearing position as soon as possible.

Practical Approach

The various drugs for treatment of hypercalcemia of malignancy are summarized in Table 3. The regimen for the therapy of hypercalcemia of malignancy depends on the level of serum calcium, the extent to which hypercalcemia is a clinical problem, and the underlying disease (Table 4). When the decision to treat hypercalcemia is made, the actions and side effects of the different drugs have to be considered with respect to the specific metabolic situation of the patient.

The first step in all patients with symptomatic hypercalcemia should be (re)hydration with saline. This is often adequate in patients with mild hyper-

Table 3. Therapy of hypercalcemia of malignancy

Therapy	Route of administration	Dosage	Onset of effect (h)	Adverse effect
Saline (0.9%)	i.v.	2–4 l over 24 h	6–12	Volume overload; hypokalemia
Calcitonin	i.v./s.c./i.m.	4–8 IU/s.c. every 6–12 h	2–6	Nausea and vomiting
Furosemide	i.v.	40–80 mg/24 h	2–4	Hypokalemia; volume depletion
Clodronate	i.v.	300 mg/day	24–48	Renal toxicity
Pamidronate	i.v.	60 mg/day	24–48	Renal toxicity
Mithramycin (plicamycin)	i.v.	25 μg/kg every 48–72 h	24	Nausea and vomiting; bleeding disorders
Prednisone	i.v.	40 mg/day	24–48	Infection; gastrointestinal bleeding

Table 4. Treatment of hypercalcemia of malignancy depending on the serum calcium concentration

Elevation of serum calcium concentration		
Mild (<3.0 mmol/l)	Moderate (<3.5 mmol/l)	Severe (>3.5 mmol/l)
	Rehydration	Rehydration Calcitonin
Hydration	Hydration and furosemide	Hydration and furosemide
	Bisphosphonate	Bisphosponate; repeat bisphosphonate; glucocorticoids; plicamycin

calcemia and no further drug therapy is required (Table 4). If hypercalcemia is more severe, sufficient rehydration is essential and a bisphosphonate is given intravenously. If symptoms are severe, the initial serum calcium level is >3.5 mol/l, or renal function is affected, intravenous calcitonin is added to the drug regimen on the first 2 days to achieve a faster decrease in serum calcium. Loop diuretics are only given to prevent overhydration in patients with cardiovascular disease. Glucocorticoids are used in addition in treating patients with hematological malignancies. Plicamycin and gallium nitrate are second- or third-line drugs to be used when repeated therapy with bisphosphonates is unsuccessful in normalization of serum calcium. As long as the therapy of the underlying malignancy is not effective, hypercalcemia can recur. In such cases temporary vigorous oral hydration and oral bisphosphonates may be useful. It is a difficult and demanding task to manage patients with hypercalcemia and advanced cancer. Besides the management of drug therapy the decision must sometimes be made to stop symptomatic calcium-lowering therapy. This is particularly true when life quality is not improved and no effective treatment for the underlying malignancy is available.

References

Attie MF (1989) Treatment of hypercalcemia. Endocrinol Metab Clin North Am 18:807–828

Bajorunas DR (1990) Clinical manifestation of cancer-related hypercalcemia. Semin Oncol 17[Suppl 5]:16–25

Benner DE, Harvey HA, Lipton A (1982) A study of prostaglandin E_2, parathormone, and response to indomethacin in patients with hypercalcemia of malignancy. Cancer 49:556–561

Bilezikian JP (1992) Management of acute hypercalcemia. N Engl J Med 326: 1196–1203

Binstock ML, Mundy GR (1980) Effect of calcitonin and glucocorticoids in combination on the hypercalcemia of malignancy. Ann Intern Med 93:269–272

Blind E, Raue F, Zisterer A, Kohl B, Ziegler R (1990) Epidemiologie der Hypercalciämie, Bedeutung der Bestimmung des intakten Parathormons für die Differentialdiagnose. Dtsch Med Wochenschr 115:1739–1745

Blind E, Raue F, Götzmann J, Schmidt-Gayk H, Kohl B, Ziegler R (1992) Circulating levels of parathyroid hormone-related protein in hypercalcemia of malignancy. Clin Endocrinol 37:290–297

Bockman RS (1991) Studies on the mechanism of action of gallium nitrate. Semin Oncol 18[suppl 5]:21–25

Body JJ, Delmas PD (1992) Urinary pyridium crosslinks as markers or bone resorption in tumor-associated hypercalcemia. J Clin Endocrinol Metab 74:471–475

Body JJ, Dumon JC, Seraj F, Cleeren A (1992) Recovery of parathyroid hormone secretion during correction of tumor-associated hypercalcemia. J Clin Endocrinol Metab 74:1385–1388

Body JJ, Dumon JC, Thirion M, Cleeren A (1993) Circulating PTHrP concentrations in tumor-induced hypercalcemia – influence on the response to bisphosphonate and changes after therapy. J Bone Miner Res 8:701–706

Bonjour JP, Rizzoli R (1992) Antiosteolytic agents in the management of hypercalcemia. Ann Oncol 3:589–590

Bonjour JP, Philippe J, Guelpa G (1988) Bone and renal components in hypercalcemia of malignancy evaluated in relation with the response to one single infusion of clodronate. Bone 9:123–130

Boonekamp PM, van der Wee-Pals LJA, van Wijk-van Lennep MML, Thesing CW, Bijvoet OLM (1988) Two modes of action of bisphosphonates on osteoclastic resorption of mineralized matrix. Bone Miner 1:27–39

Bounameaux HM, Schifferli J, Jung A, Chatelant F (1983) Renal failure with intravenous bisphosphonates. Lancet 1:471

Breslau NA, McGuire JL, Zerwekh JE, Frenkel EP, Pak CYC (1984) Hypercalcemia associated with increased serum calcitriol levels in three patients with lymphoma. Ann Intern Med 100:1–7

Brown JH, Kennedy BJ (1965) Mithramycin in the treatment of testicular cancer. N Engl J Med 272:111–118

Bunn A, Schechter GP, Jaffe ES, Blaney D, Young RC, Mathews MJ, Blattner W, Broder S, Robert-Guroff M, Gallo RC (1983) Clinical course of retrovirus-

associated adult T-cell lymphoma in the United States. N Engl J Med 309:257–264
Cardella CJ, Birkin BL, Rapoport A (1979) Role of dialysis in the treatment of severe hypercalcemia: report of two cases successfully treated with hemodialysis and review of the literature. clin Nephrol 12:285–290
Chabner BA (1993) Anticancer drugs. In: DeVita VT, Hellmann S, Rosenberg SA (eds) Cancer – principles and practice of oncology Lippincott, Philadelphia, pp 325–340
Conlin PR, Fajtova VT, Mortensen RM, LeBoff MS, Brown EM (1989) Hysteresis in the relationship between serum ionized calcium and intact parathyroid hormone during recovery from induced hyper- and hypocalcemia in normal humans. J Clin Endocrinol Metab 69:593–599
Coombs RC, Ward MK, Greenberg PB (1976) Calcium metabolism in cancer studies using calcium isotopes and immunoassays for parathyroid hormones and calcitonin. Cancer 38:2111–2116
De Vernejoul MC, Pointillart A, Bergot C, Bielakoff J, Morieux C, Laval Jantet AM, Miravet L (1987) Different schedules of administration of (3-amino-1-hydroxypropylidene)-1,1-bisphosphonate induce different changes in pig bone remodelling. Calcif Tissue Int 40:160–165
Delmas PD, Demioux B, Malaval L (1986) Serum bone gamma-carboxyglutamic acid-containing protein in primary hyperparathyroidism and in malignant hypercalcemia. J Clin Invest 77:985–991
Dodwell DJ, Abbas SK, Morton AR, Howell A (1991) Parathyroid hormone-related protein (50–69) and response to pamidronate therapy of tumour-induced hypercalcemia. Eur J Cancer 27:1629–1633
Douglas DL, Kanis JA, Paterson AD, Beard DJ, Cameron EC, Watson ME, Woodhead S, Williams J, Russell RGG (1983) Drug treatment of primary hyperparathroidism: use of clodronate disodium. Br Med J 286:587–590
Dumon JC, Magritte A, Body JJ (1991) Efficacy and safety of the bisphosphonate tiludronate for the treatment of the tumor-associated hypercalcemia. Bone Miner 15:257–266
Dumon JC, Magritte A, Body JJ (1992) Nasal human calcitonin for tumor-induced hypercalcemia. Calcif Tissue Int 51:18–19
Eilon G, Mundy G (1978) Direct resorption of bone by human breast cancer cells in vitro. Nature 276:726–728
Elomaa I, Blomqvist C, Grohn P, Porkka L, Kairento AL, Selander K, Lamberg-Allardt C, Holmstrom T (1983) Long term controlled trial with diphosphonate in patients with osteolytic bone metastases. Lancet 1:146–149
Evans RA, Howlett CR, Dunstan CR, Hills E (1982) The effect of long-term low dose diphosphonate treatment on rat bone. Clin Orthop Res 165:290–299
Fatemi S, Singer FR, Rude RK (1992) Effect of salmon calcitonin and etidronate on hypercalcemia of malignancy. Calcif Tissue Int 50:107–109
Flanagan AM, Chambers TJ (1989) Dichloromethylenebisphosphonate (Cl_2 MBP) inhibits bone resorption through injury to osteoclasts that resorb Cl_2 MBP coated bone. Bone Miner 6:33–43
Fleisch H (1989) Bisphosphonates: a new class of drugs in diseases of bone and calcium metabolism. In: Brunner KW, Fleisch H, Senn HJ (eds) Bisphosphonates and tumor osteolysis. Springer, Berlin Heibelberg New York, pp 1–28
Fleisch H (1991) Bisphosphonates – pharmacology and use in treatment of tumour-induced hypercalcemia and metastatic bone disease. Drugs 42:919–944
Fogelman I, McKillop JH (1991) The bone scan in metastatic disease. In: Rubens RD, Fogelman I (eds) Bone metastases – diagnosis and treatment. Springer, Berlin Heidelberg New York, pp 32–61

Frijlink WB, Bijvoet OLM, te Velde J, Heynen G (1979) Treatment of Paget's disease with (3-amino-1-hydroxypropylidene)-1,1-bisphosphonate (APD). Lancet 1:799–803

Garrett IR, Durie BGM, Glenn EN, Gillespie A, Bringman T, Sabatini M, Bertolini DR, Mundy GR (1987) Production of lymphotoxin, a bone resorbing cytokine, by cultured human myeloma cells. N Engl J Med 317:526–549

Glover DJ, Riley L, Carmichael K, Spar B, Glick J, Kligerman MM, Agus ZA, Slatopolsky E, Attie M, Goldfarb S (1983) Hypocalcemia and inhibition of parathyroid hormone secretion after administration of WR-2721 (a radioprotective and chemoprotective agent). N Engl J Med 309:1137–1141

Glover DJ, Shaw L, Glick JH, Slatopolsky E, Weiler C, Attie M, Goldfarb S (1985) Treatment of hypercalcemia in parathyroid cancer with WR-2721, S-2-(3-aminopaopylamino) ethyl-phosphorothioic acid. Ann Intern Med 103:55–57

Greaves M, Ibbotson J, Atkins D, Martin TJ (1980) Prostaglandins as mediators of bone resorption in renal and breast tumours. Clin Sci 58:201–210

Grill V, Murray RML, Ho PWM, Santamaria JD, Pitt P, Potts C, Jerums G, Martin TJ (1992) Circulating PTH and PTHrP levels before and after treatment of tumor induced hypercalcemia with pamidronate disodium (APD). J Clin Endocrinol Metab 74:1468–1471

Gucalp R, Ritch P, Wiernik PH, Sarma PR, Keller A, Richman SP, Tauer K, Neidhart J, Malette LE, Siegel R, Vandepol CJ (1992) Comparative study of pamidronate disodium and etidronate disodium in the treatment of cancer-related hypercalcemia. J Clin Oncol 10:134–142

Guidon PT, Salvatori R, Bockmann RS (1993) Gallium nitrate regulates rat osteoblast expression of osteocalcin protein and mRNA levels. J Bone Miner Res 8:103–112

Guncage J, Lauffenburger R, Lentner C, Dambacher MA, Haas HG, Fleisch H, Olah AJ (1974) Diphosphonate treatment of Paget's disease of bone. A correlated metabolic, calcium kinetic and morphometric study. Horm Metab Res 6:62–69

Gurney H, Kefford R, Strart-Harris R (1989) Renal phosphate threshold and respose to pamidronate in humoral hypercalcemia of malignancy. Lancet 2:241–244

Gurney H, Grill V, Martin TJ (1993) Parathyroid hormone-related protein and response to pamidronate in tumour-induced hypercalcaemia. Lancet 341: 1611–1613

Harinck HLJ, Bijvoet OLM, Platingh AST, Body II, Elte JWF, Sleebom HP, Wildiers J, Neijt JP (1987) Role of bone and kidney in tumor-induduced hyperalcemia and its treatment with bisphosphonate and sodium cloride, Am J Med 82:1133–1142

Hosking DJ, Gilson D (1984) Comparison of the renal and skeletal actions of calcitonin in the treatment of severe hypercalcemia of malignancy. Q J Med 53:359–368

Hosking DJ, Cowley A, Bucknall CA (1981) Rehydration in the treatment of severe hypercalcemia. Q J Med 50:473–481

Hosking DJ, Stone MD, Foote JW (1990) Potentiation of calcitonin by corticosteroids during the treatment of the hypercalcemia of malignancy. Eur J Clin Pharmacol 38:37–41

Ibbotson KJ, D'Souza SM, Smith DD, Carpenter G, Mundy GR (1985) EGF receptor antiserum inhibits the bone resorbing activity produced by a rat Leydig cell tumour associated with the humoral hypercalcemia of cancer. Endocrinology 116:469–476

Ikeda K, Lu C, Weir EC, Mangin M, Broadus AE (1989) Transcriptional regulation of the parathyroid hormone-related peptide gene by glucocorticoids and vitamin D in a human C-cell line. J Biol Chem 264:15743–15746

Jacobs TP, Siris ES, Bilezikian JP, Bagurian DC, Shane E, Canfield RE (1981) Hypercalcemia of malignancy: treatment with intravenous dichloromethylene diphosphonate. Ann Intern Med 94:312–316
Kanis JA, McCloskey EV, Paterson AHG (1990) Use of diphosphonates in hypercalcemia due to malignancy. Lancet 1:170–171
Kasono K, Isozaki O, Sato K, Sato Y, Shizume K, Ohsumi K, Demura H (1991) Effects of glucocorticoids and calcitonin on parathyroid hormone-related protein (PTHrP) gene expession and PTHrP release in human cancer cells causing humoral hypercalcemia. Jpn J Med 82:1008–1014
Lu C, Ikeda K, Deftos LJ, Gazdar AF, Mangin M, Broadus AE (1989) Glucocorticoid regulation of parathyroid hormone-related peptide gene transcription in a human neuroendocrine cell line. Mol Endocrinol 3:2034–2040
Marie PJ, Hott M, Garba MT (1985) Inhibition of bone matrix apposition by (3-amino-1-hydroxypropylidene)-1,1,-bisphosphonate (AHPrBP) in the mouse. Bone 6:193–200
Marshall MJ, Wilson AS, Davie MWJ (1990) Effects of (3-amino-1-hydroxypropylidene)-1,1-bisphosphonate on mouse osteoclasts. J Bone Miner Res 5:955–962
Martin TJ, Grill V (1992) Hypercalcemia in cancer. J Steroid Biochem Mol Biol. 43:123–129
Miller SC, Jee WSS, Kimmel DB, Woodbury L (1977) Ethane-1-hydroxy-1,1-diphosphonate (EHDP) effects on incorporation and accumulation of osteoclast nuclei. Calcif Tissue Res 22:243–252
Mosekilde L, Charles P, Lindegreen P (1989) Determinants of serum 1,25-dihydroxycholecalciferol in primary hyperparathyroidism. Bone Miner 5:279–285
Moskilde L, Fink E, Charles P (1991) Hypercalcemia of maligmancy: pathophysiology, diagnosis and treatment. Crit Rev Oncol Hematol 11:1–27
Motokura T, Fukumoto S, Matsumoto T, Takahashi S, Fujita A, Yamashita T, Igarashi T, Ogata E (1989) Parathyroid hormone-related protein in adult T-cell leukemia-lymphoma. Ann Intern Med 111:484–488
Mühlbauer RC, Bauss F, Schenk R, Janner M, Bosies E, Strein K, Fleisch H (1991) BM 21.0955, a potent new bisphosphonate to inhibit bone resorption. J Bone Miner Res 6:1003–1011
Mundy GR (1990a) Hypercalcemia associated with hematological maligncies. In: Mundy GR (ed) Calcium homeostasis: hypercalcemia and hypocalcemia. Dunitz, London, pp 100–116
Mundy GR (1990b) Treatment of hypercalcemia due to malignancy. In: Mundy GR (ed) Calcium homeostasis: hypercalcemia and hypocalcemia. Dunitz, London, pp 117–138
Mundy GR, Martin TJ (1992) Hypercalcemia of malignancy: pathogenesis and management. Metabolism 31:1247–1277
Mundy GR, Wilkinson R, Heath DA (1983) Comparative study of available medical therapy for hypercalcemia of malignancy. Am J Med 74:421–432
Nussbaum SR, Zahradnik RJ, Lavigne JR, Brennan K, Nozaw-Ung K, Kim LY, Keutmann HT, Wand CA, Potts JT, Segre GV (1987) Highly sensitive two-site immuno radiometric assay of parathyrin, and its clinical utility in evaluating patients with hypercalcemia. Clin Chem 33:1364–1369
O'Rourke NP, McCloskey EV, Vasikaran S, Eyres K, Fem D, Kanis JA (1993) Effective treatment of malignant hypercalcemia with a single intravenous infusion of clodronate Br J Cancer 67:560–563
Papapoulos SE, Harinck HIJ, Bijvoet OLM, Gleed JH, Fraher LJ, O'Riordan JLH (1986) Effect of decreasing serum calcium on circulating parathyroid hormone and vitamin D metabolites in normocalcemic and hypercalcemic patients treated with APD. Bone Miner 1:69–78

Paterson AD, Kanis JA, Cameron EC, Douglas DL, Beard DJ, Preston FE, Russell RGG (1983) The use of dichloromethylene diphosphonate for the management of hypercalcemia in multiple myeloma. Br J Haematol 54:121–132
Pecherstorfer M, Thièbaud D (1992) Treatment of resistant tumor-induced hypercalcemia with escalating doses of pamidronate (APD). Ann Oncol 3:661–663
Pecherstorfer M, Janisch S, Marosi C, Wogritsch C, Bosse C, Schratzberger W, Gerber E, Fortelny A, Lenzhofer R, Rainer H, Klaushofer K, Baumgartner G, Schernthaner G (1991) Treatment of cancer associated-hypercalcemia with pamidronate. Klin Wochenschr 69:690–695
Pecherstorfer M, Schilling T, Blind E, Baumgartner G (1992) Influence of bisphosphonate treatment of parathyroid hormone (PTH) and parathyroid hormone-related protein (PTHrP) Proc Am Assoc Cancer Res 33:284
Pecherstorfer M, Schilling T, Janisch S, Woloszczuk W, Baumgartner G, Ziegler R, Ogris E (1993c) Effect of clodronate treatment on bone scintigraphy in metastatic breast cancer. J Nucl Med 34:1039–1044
Pecherstorfer M, Seibel MJ, Zimmer-Roth I, Schilling T, Baumgartner G (1993b) Effect of bisphosphonate therapy on urinary pyridinium crosslinks in tumor associated hypercalcemia. Proc Am Soc Clin Oncol 12:112
Pecherstorfer M, Jilch R, Zimmer-Roth I, Sauty A, Baumgartner G, Thièbaud D (1993c) The osteoclast inhibitor pamidronate increases serum levels of tumor necrosis factor α and enhances expression of early activation markers. Proc Am Assoc Cancer Res 34:221
Percival RC, Yates AJP, Gray RES, Neal FE, Forrest ARW, Kanis JA (1984) Role of glucocorticoids in the management of malignant hypercalcemia. Br Med J 200:204–209
Percival RC, Yates AJP, Gray RES, Galloway J, Rogers K, Neal FE, Kanis JA (1985) Mechanisms of malignant hypercalcemia in carcinoma of the breast. Br Med J 291:776–779
Powell GJ, Southby J, Danks JA, Stillwell RG, Hayman JA, Henderson MA, Bennett RC, Martin TJ (1991) Localization of parathyroid hormone related protein in breast cancer metastases: increased incidence in bone compared with other sites. Cancer Res 51:3959–3961
Raisz LG, Trummel CL, Weiner JA (1972) Effect of glucocorticoids on bone resorption in tissue culture. Endocrinology 90:961–967
Ralston SH, Fogelman I, Gardner MD (1984) Hypercalcemia of malignancy: evidence for a non-parathyroid humoral agent with an effect on renal tubular calcium handling. Clin Sci 66:187–191
Ralston SH, Gardner MD, Dryburgh FJ, Jenkins AS, Cowan RA, Boyle IT (1985) Comparison of aminohydroxypropylidene diphosphate, mithramycin, and corticosteroids/calcitonin in treatment of cancer-associated hypercalcemia. Lancet 2:907–910
Ralston H, Gallagher SJ, Patel U, Dryburgh FJ, Fraser W, Cowan RA, Boyle IT (1989) Comparison of three intravenous bisphosphonates in cancer-associated hypercalcemia. Lancet 2:1180–1182
Ralston SH, Gallacher SJ, Patel U, Campbell J, Boyle IT (1990) Cancer-associated hypercalcemia: morbidity and mortality. Ann Intern Med 112:499–504
Reiner M, Sautter V, Olah A, Bossi A, Largiadèr U, Fleisch H (1980) Diphosphonate treatment in myositis ossificans progressiva. In: Cannigia A (ed.) Etidronate. Instituto Gentili, Pisa, p 237
Ritch PS (1990) Treatment of cancer-related hypercalcemia. Semin Oncol 17[Suppl 5]:26–39

Rosenthal N, Insogna KL, Godsall JW, Smaldone L, Waldron JA, Stewart AF (1985) Elevations in circulating 1,25-dihydroxyvitamin D in three patients with lymphoma associated hypercalcemia. Clin Endocrinol Metab 60:29–33

Rosol TJ, Capen CC (1992) Biology of disease – mechanisms of cancer-induced hypercalcemia. Lab Invest 67:680–702

Russell RGG, Smith R, Preston C, Walton RJ, Woods CG (1974) Diphosphonates in Paget's disease. Lancet 1:894–898

Schilling T, Pecherstorfer M, Blind E, Leidig G, Ziegler R, Raue F (1993) Parathyroid hormone-related protein (PTHrP) does not regulate 1,25-dihydroxyvitamin D serum levels in hypercalcemia of malignancy. J Clin Endocrinol Metab 76:801–803

Seyberth HW, Segre GV, Morgasn JL, Sweetman BJ, Potts JT, Oates JA (1975) Prostaglandins as mediators of hypercalcemia associated with certain types of cancer. N Engl J Med 293:1278–1283

Shackney S, Hasson J (1967) Precipitous fall in serum calcium, hypotension, and acute renal failure after intravenous phosphate therapy for hypercalcemia: report of two cases. Ann Intern Med 66:906–916

Shane E (1990) Hypercalcemia: differential diagnosis and management. In: Favus MJ (ed) Primer on metabolic bone disease. ASBMR, pp 107–108

Shirakawa F, Yamashita U, Tanaka Y, Watanaba K, Sato K, Haratake J, Fujihira T, Oda S, Eto S (1988) Production of bone-resorbing activity corresponding to interleukin-1α by adult T-cell leukemia cells in humans. Cancer Res 48:4284–4287

Silva OL, Becker KL (1973) Salmon calcitonin in the treatment of hypercalcemia. Arch Intern Med 132:337–339

Singer FR (1991) Pathogenesis of hypercalcemia of malignancy. Semin Oncol 18:4–10

Stewart AF, Horst R, Deftos LJ, Cadman EC, Lang R, Broadus AE (1980) Biochemical evaluation of patients with cancer-associated hypercalcemia: evidence for humoral and nonhumoral groups. N Engl J Med 303:1377–1383

Suki WN, Yium JJ, von Minden M, Saller-Herbert C, Eknovan G, Martinez-Maldonado M (1970) Acute treatment of hypercalcemia with furosemide. N Engl J Med 283:836–840

Thiébaud D, Jaeger P, Jacquet AF, Burckhardt P (1988) Dose-response in the treatment of hypercalcemia of malignancy by a single infusion of the bisphosphonate AHPrBP. J Clin Oncol 6:762–768

Thiébaud D, Jaeger P, Burckhardt P (1990) Response to retreatment of malignant hypercalcemia with the bisphosphonate AHPrBP (APD): respective role of kidney and one. J Bone Miner Res 5:221–225

Thürlimann B, Waldburger R, Senn HJ, Thiéboud D (1992) Plicamycin and pamidronate in symptomatic tumor related-hypercalcemia: a prospective randomized cross over trial. Ann Oncel 3:619–623

Todd PA, Fitton A (1991) Gallium nitrate, a review of its pharmacological properties and therapeutic potential in cancer-related hypercalcemia. Drugs 42:261–273

Vernava AM, O'Neal LW, Palermo V (1987) Lethal hyperparathyroid crisis: hazard of phosphate administration. Surgery 102:941–948

Warrell PR (1993) Metabolic emergencies – hypercalcemia. In: DeVita VT, Hellmann S, Rosenberg SA (eds) Cancer – principles and practice of oncoloy. Lippincott, Philadelphia, pp 2128–2142

Warrell RP, Skelos A, Alcock NW (1986) Gallium nitrate for acute treatment of cancer-related hypercalcemia: clinicopharmacological and dose response analysis. Cancer Res 46:4208–4212

Warrell RP, Alcock NW, Bockman RS (1987) Gallium nitrate inhibits accelerated bone turnover in patients with bone metastases. J Clin Oncol 5:292–298
Warrell RP, Israel R, Frisone M, Snyder T, Gaynor JJ, Bockman RS (1988) Gallium nitrate for acute treatment of cancer-related hypercalcemia: a randomized, double-blind comparison to calcitonin. Ann Intern Med 108:669–674
Warrell RP, Murphy WP, Schulman P (1991) A randomized double-blind study of gallium nitrate compared to etidronate for acute control of cancer-related hypercalcemia. J Clin Oncol 9:1467–1475
Wisneski LA (1990) Salmon calcitonin in the acute management of hypercalcemia. Calcif Tissue Int 46:S26–S30
Yabro JW, Kennedy BJ, Barnum CP (1965) Mithramycin inhibition of ribonucleic acid synthesis. Cancer Res 26:36–39
Ziegler R, Scharla SH (1989) Treatment of tumor hypercalcemia with clodronate. In: Brunner KW, Fleisch H, Senn HJ (eds) Bisphosphonates and tumor ostelysis. Springer, Berlin Heidelberg New York, pp 46–53 (Recent results cancer research, vol 116)
Zysset E, Ammann P, Jezer A, Gertz BJ, Portmann L, Rizzoli R, Jaquet-miiller F, Pryor-Tillotson S, Bonjour JP, Burckhardt P (1992) Comparison of a rapid (2-h) versus a slow (24 h) infusion of alendronate in the treatment of hyperculcemia of malignancy. Bone Miner 18:237–249

Subject Index

Springer-Verlag and the Environment

We at Springer-Verlag firmly believe that an international science publisher has a special obligation to the environment, and our corporate policies consistently reflect this conviction.

We also expect our business partners – paper mills, printers, packaging manufacturers, etc. – to commit themselves to using environmentally friendly materials and production processes.

The paper in this book is made from low- or no-chlorine pulp and is acid free, in conformance with international standards for paper permanency.

MIX
Papier aus verantwortungsvollen Quellen
Paper from responsible sources
FSC® C105338

If you have any concerns about our products,
you can contact us on
ProductSafety@springernature.com

In case Publisher is established outside the EU,
the EU authorized representative is:
Springer Nature Customer Service Center GmbH
Europaplatz 3, 69115 Heidelberg, Germany

Printed by Libri Plureos GmbH
in Hamburg, Germany